COOKBOOK
TABLE OF CONTENTS

INTRODUCTION

About Noom	2
Noom's Dietary Guidelines	4
Food Category	8
Menu templates for breakfast, lunch, dinner and snacks.	11

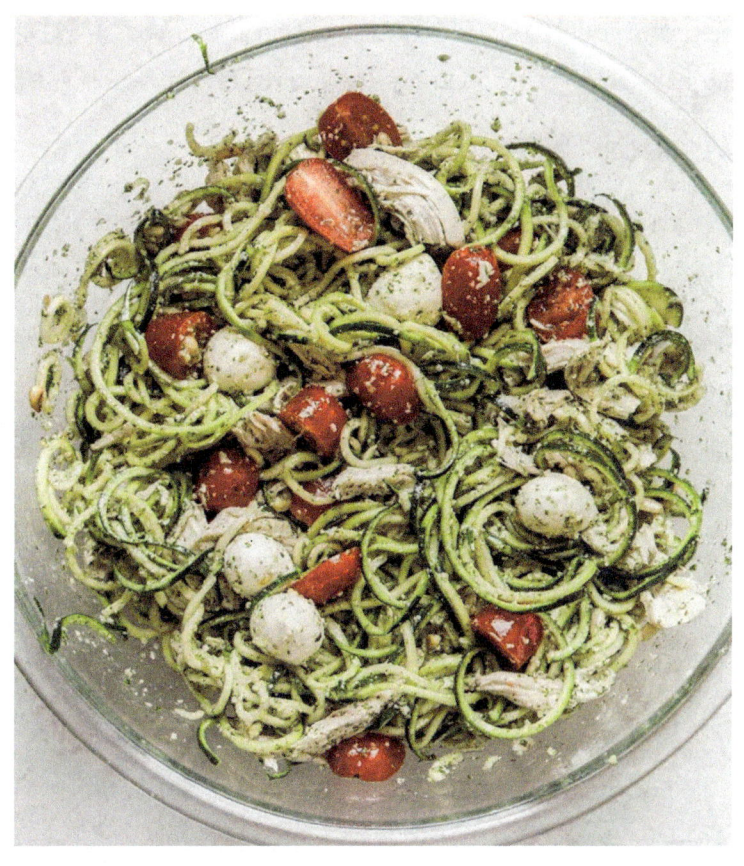

CHAPTER 01 — 12
Breakfast

CHAPTER 02 — 32
Lunch

CHAPTER 03 — 52
Afternoon Snack

CHAPTER 04 — 74
Dinner

CHAPTER 05 — 115
Desserts

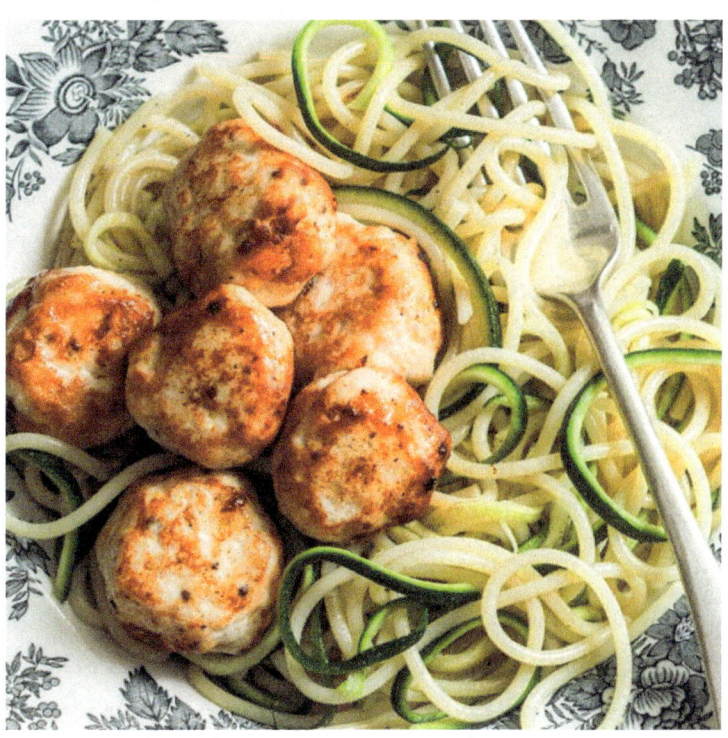

ABOUT NOOM

Overview of Noom and Its Weight Loss Method

Noom is a revolutionary weight loss program that combines cutting-edge technology with behavioral psychology to help individuals achieve and maintain their weight loss goals. Unlike traditional diets that focus solely on food and exercise, Noom emphasizes the mental and emotional aspects of weight management.

What is Noom?

Noom is a mobile app-based weight loss program that uses a personalized approach to help users make lasting changes in their eating habits and lifestyle. The program is designed to address the psychological factors that contribute to weight gain and support users in developing healthier behaviors.

Core Principles of Noom:

1. **Behavioral Psychology:** Noom incorporates principles from cognitive-behavioral therapy (CBT) to help users understand and modify their eating behaviors. The program focuses on changing thought patterns and habits that lead to overeating and weight gain.
2. **Calorie Density:** The diet emphasizes eating foods that are low in calorie density but high in nutrients. By focusing on foods that are filling and nutritious, users can eat larger portions without consuming excessive calories.
3. **Food Categorization:** Noom categorizes foods into three color groups: green, yellow, and red. Green foods are low in calories and high in nutrients, yellow foods have moderate calorie content, and red foods are higher in calories and should be consumed in moderation. This system helps users make informed choices about their food.
4. **Personalized Coaching:** Users receive support from personal health coaches who provide guidance, encouragement, and accountability. Coaches help users set realistic goals, overcome obstacles, and stay motivated throughout their weight loss journey.
5. **Tracking and Insights:** The Noom app offers tools for tracking food intake, physical activity, and progress. It also provides personalized insights and recommendations based on users' data, helping them stay on track and make informed decisions.

Why Noom is Effective:

Focus on Behavior Change: By addressing the psychological aspects of weight loss, Noom helps users build sustainable habits and create lasting changes in their lifestyle.

Personalization: The program's individualized approach ensures that recommendations and strategies are tailored to each user's unique needs and goals.

Holistic Approach: Noom combines nutrition, exercise, and mental health to provide a comprehensive weight management solution that goes beyond traditional dieting methods.

Explanation of Noom's Food Classification System (Green, Yellow, Red)

Noom's food classification system is a core component of its weight loss program, designed to simplify food choices and support healthy eating habits. The system categorizes foods into three color groups—green, yellow, and red—based on their calorie density and nutritional value. Here's a detailed explanation of each category:

Green Foods

- **Definition:** Foods in the green category are low in calorie density and high in essential nutrients. These foods are typically rich in vitamins, minerals, and fiber, while being low in calories.
- **Examples:** Leafy greens (spinach, kale), vegetables (broccoli, bell peppers), fruits (berries, apples), legumes (beans, lentils).
- **Benefits:** Green foods are filling and nutritious, allowing you to eat larger portions without consuming too many calories. They help promote satiety and support overall health and well-being.
- **Recommendations:** Incorporate green foods into every meal to ensure a high intake of nutrients while keeping calorie consumption in check.

Yellow Foods

- **Definition:** Yellow foods have a moderate calorie density and provide a balance between calories and nutritional value. They include foods that are more calorie-dense than green foods but still offer important nutrients.
- **Examples:** Fruits (bananas, oranges), whole grains (brown rice, oats), lean proteins (chicken breast, tofu), starchy vegetables (sweet potatoes, corn).
- **Benefits:** While these foods provide essential nutrients and energy, it's important to consume them in controlled portions to manage calorie intake.
- **Recommendations:** Use yellow foods to add variety and balance to your diet. Pay attention to portion sizes to avoid consuming excess calories.

Red Foods

- **Definition:** Red foods are higher in calorie density and often contain more fats, sugars, or refined ingredients. These foods are typically more calorie-dense and less nutrient-dense compared to green and yellow foods.
- **Examples:** Processed snacks (chips, cookies), sugary beverages (soda, fruit juices), high-fat meats (bacon, sausage), desserts (cakes, pastries).
- **Benefits:** Red foods can be enjoyed in moderation but should not be a staple in your diet. They are often higher in calories and less filling, which can lead to overeating if consumed in large amounts.
- **Recommendations:** Limit the intake of red foods and enjoy them occasionally. Focus on moderation and portion control to prevent excess calorie consumption.

Overall Guidance

- **Balance and Moderation:** The key to using Noom's food classification system effectively is to balance your intake of green, yellow, and red foods. The majority of your diet should consist of green foods, with controlled portions of yellow foods and limited consumption of red foods.
- **Informed Choices:** The color-coded system helps you make informed choices about what to eat, guiding you toward healthier options while allowing flexibility in your diet.

NOOM'S DIETARY GUIDELINES

Introduction to Noom's Eating Principles and How to Apply Them in Practice

Noom's eating principles focus on fostering a balanced and sustainable approach to nutrition by integrating behavioral psychology with dietary guidelines. These principles are designed to help individuals make healthier food choices, build lasting habits, and achieve their weight loss goals. Here's a detailed look at Noom's eating principles and practical ways to apply them:

Core Principles of Noom's Eating Approach

Behavioral Psychology Integration

- Focus on Mindset: Noom emphasizes the importance of changing your mindset and behavior toward food. It helps you recognize and alter patterns of thinking that lead to unhealthy eating habits.
- Self-Awareness: By understanding your triggers for overeating and emotional eating, you can develop strategies to manage these behaviors and make more mindful food choices.

Calorie Density Concept

- Understanding Calorie Density: Noom teaches that foods vary in calorie density, which is the number of calories per unit of weight. Foods with low calorie density, like vegetables and fruits, provide more volume and satiety for fewer calories.
- Application: Focus on incorporating low-calorie-density foods (green foods) into your meals to help you feel full while managing your calorie intake.

Food Categorization System

- Green, Yellow, and Red Foods: Noom categorizes foods into three color groups based on their calorie density and nutritional value.
    - Green Foods: Low in calories, high in nutrients. Aim to fill most of your plate with these foods.
    - Yellow Foods: Moderately calorie-dense, providing essential nutrients. Consume these in controlled portions.
    - Red Foods: High in calories and less nutrient-dense. Limit these foods and consume them in moderation.
- Application: Use this system to guide your food choices and create a balanced plate. Prioritize green foods, balance yellow foods, and enjoy red foods sparingly.

NOOM'S DIETARY GUIDELINES

Mindful Eating Practices

- **Listening to Your Body:** Pay attention to your body's hunger and fullness cues to avoid overeating. Eat when you are truly hungry and stop when you are satisfied.
- **Eating Slowly:** Take your time to savor each bite and enjoy your meal. Eating slowly helps you recognize when you are full and reduces the risk of overeating.
- **Practical Tips:** Use smaller plates, chew thoroughly, and avoid distractions (like TV or smartphones) while eating.

Portion Control

- **Understanding Portions:** Noom teaches you to manage portion sizes to prevent overeating. Learn to gauge appropriate portion sizes and use visual cues to help control your intake.
- **Application:** Use tools like measuring cups or a food scale to help you understand and control portion sizes. Pay attention to serving sizes listed on food labels.

Personalized Goals and Tracking

- **Setting Realistic Goals:** Noom encourages setting specific, measurable, achievable, relevant, and time-bound (SMART) goals for your eating habits and weight loss.
- **Tracking Progress:** Utilize Noom's app to track your food intake, physical activity, and progress. Regular tracking helps you stay accountable and adjust your habits as needed.
- **Application:** Use the app's tracking features to monitor your meals and progress. Reflect on your goals and adjust your strategies based on your tracking data.

Applying Noom's Principles in Daily Life

1. **Plan Your Meals:** Use Noom's food categorization and portion control principles to plan balanced meals. Incorporate a variety of green and yellow foods into your daily eating routine, and be mindful of red food consumption.
2. **Prepare Your Environment:** Create a supportive environment by stocking your kitchen with healthy green and yellow foods, and limiting the availability of red foods.
3. **Practice Mindfulness:** Incorporate mindful eating practices into your daily routine. Take time to enjoy your meals and recognize your body's hunger and fullness signals.
4. **Stay Engaged with Noom:** Regularly interact with Noom's app, engage with your health coach, and utilize the resources provided to stay on track with your weight loss journey.

NOOM'S DIETARY GUIDELINES

Tips for Choosing Foods Based on Noom's Color System

Noom's color-coding system helps simplify food choices by categorizing foods into three groups: green, yellow, and red. Each category represents different calorie densities and nutritional values, guiding you to make healthier decisions. Here are some practical tips for choosing foods based on this system:

1. **Prioritize Green Foods**
   - **Focus on Nutrient-Rich Options:** Green foods are low in calories but high in essential nutrients. Aim to fill the majority of your plate with these foods to maximize nutrition while managing calorie intake.
     - **Examples:** Leafy greens (spinach, kale), non-starchy vegetables (broccoli, bell peppers), fruits (berries, apples), and legumes (beans, lentils).
   - **Meal Ideas:** Create salads with a variety of vegetables, add spinach or kale to smoothies, and enjoy large servings of roasted or steamed vegetables.

2. **Use Yellow Foods in Moderation**
   - **Balance Your Meals:** Yellow foods are moderately calorie-dense, offering a balance between nutrients and calories. Use these foods to add variety and flavor to your meals, but be mindful of portion sizes.
     - **Examples:** Fruits (bananas, oranges), whole grains (brown rice, quinoa), lean proteins (chicken breast, tofu), and starchy vegetables (sweet potatoes, corn).
   - **Meal Ideas:** Include a serving of whole grains or a piece of fruit in your meals, and add lean proteins or starchy vegetables to complement green foods.

3. **Limit Red Foods**
   - **Consume Sparingly:** Red foods are higher in calories and often lower in nutrients. Limit your intake of these foods to avoid excessive calorie consumption and focus on moderation.
     - **Examples:** Processed snacks (chips, cookies), sugary beverages (soda, fruit juices), high-fat meats (bacon, sausage), and desserts (cakes, pastries).
   - **Meal Ideas:** Treat yourself to red foods occasionally and in small portions. For example, enjoy a small piece of dessert or a few chips as an occasional treat rather than a regular part of your diet.

NOOM'S DIETARY GUIDELINES

4. Plan Balanced Meals

- **Create a Colorful Plate:** Aim to have a balance of green, yellow, and red foods on your plate, with a focus on green foods. This approach ensures you get a variety of nutrients while keeping your calorie intake in check.
- **Meal Planning:** When planning meals, consider using green foods as the base, yellow foods to add variety and energy, and red foods as occasional additions.

5. Read Labels and Portions

- **Check Food Labels:** When choosing packaged foods, read nutrition labels to understand the calorie content and nutritional value. Opt for options that fit within the green and yellow categories.
- **Control Portions:** Be mindful of portion sizes for yellow and red foods. Use measuring tools or visual cues to help manage portion sizes and prevent overeating.

6. Be Flexible and Adapt

- **Adjust Based on Needs:** Adapt the color system to fit your individual dietary needs and preferences. If you have specific health goals or dietary restrictions, adjust your choices while still following the general principles of the color system.
- **Experiment with Recipes:** Try new recipes that incorporate a mix of green and yellow foods. Explore different ways to prepare and enjoy these foods to keep your diet varied and enjoyable.

FOOD CATEGORY

Food Classification by Color and Usage Guidelines

Noom's color-coded system categorizes foods into three groups: green, yellow, and red. Each group represents different calorie densities and nutritional values, helping you make healthier food choices. Here's a breakdown of each category and how to use them in your diet:

1. Green Foods
  - **Characteristics:** Green foods are low in calorie density and high in nutrients. They are typically rich in vitamins, minerals, and fiber, which help you feel full and satisfied with fewer calories.
  - **Examples:**
    - **Leafy Greens:** Spinach, kale, lettuce.
    - **Non-Starchy Vegetables:** Broccoli, bell peppers, cucumbers.
    - **Fruits:** Strawberries, apples, kiwi.
    - **Legumes:** Green beans, kidney beans, lentils.
  - **Usage Guidelines:**
    - **Main Meals:** Use green vegetables and non-starchy vegetables as the base of your meals. Add them to salads, soups, or stir-fries.
    - **Snacks:** Enjoy fresh fruits or cut vegetables as healthy snacks.
    - **Smoothies and Juices:** Add leafy greens to smoothies for an extra nutrient boost without adding many calories.

2. Yellow Foods
  - **Characteristics:** Yellow foods have a moderate calorie density, providing a balance between calories and nutrients. They include foods that are more calorie-dense than green foods but still offer important nutrients.
  - **Examples:**
    - **Fruits:** Bananas, oranges, apples.
    - **Whole Grains:** Brown rice, oats, quinoa.
    - **Lean Proteins:** Chicken breast, tofu, fish.
    - **Starchy Vegetables:** Sweet potatoes, corn.
  - **Usage Guidelines:**
    - **Main Meals:** Combine yellow foods with green foods to create balanced meals. For example, serve grilled chicken with a side of vegetables and sweet potatoes.
    - **Snacks:** Include fruits or whole grains in your snacks, such as a piece of fruit or a small serving of oatmeal.
    - **Special Dishes:** Use whole grains and lean proteins to provide sustained energy and balance in your meals.

FOOD CATEGORY

3. Red Foods

- **Characteristics:** Red foods are higher in calorie density and often contain more fats, sugars, or refined ingredients. They are less nutrient-dense compared to green and yellow foods.
- **Examples:**
  - **Processed Snacks:** Chips, cookies, candy.
  - **Sugary Beverages:** Soda, fruit juices with added sugar.
  - **High-Fat Meats:** Bacon, sausage.
  - **Desserts:** Cakes, pastries, ice cream.
- **Usage Guidelines:**
  - **Moderation:** Limit your intake of red foods and consume them occasionally to avoid excessive calorie consumption.
  - **Combination with Green Foods:** When you do eat red foods, balance them with green and yellow foods to create a more nutritious meal.
  - **Smart Choices:** If you indulge in red foods, choose lower-calorie versions or control portion sizes to manage calorie intake.

Summary

- **Main Meals:** Base your meals around green foods, mix in yellow foods for variety, and limit red foods to occasional treats.
- **Snacks:** Opt for green and yellow foods as healthy snacks.
- **Meal Planning:** Plan meals with a balanced mix of green, yellow, and red foods to maintain a nutritious and calorie-conscious diet.

FOOD CATEGORY

List of Green, Yellow, and Red Foods

Here is a list of foods categorized by Noom's color-coding system: green (healthy foods), yellow (moderate foods), and red (limit foods).

1. Green Foods
   - **Leafy Greens:** Spinach, kale, Swiss chard, lettuce.
   - **Non-Starchy Vegetables:** Broccoli, bell peppers, cucumbers, tomatoes, mushrooms.
   - **Fruits:** Strawberries, apples, kiwi, avocados, lemons.
   - **Legumes:** Green beans, lentils, kidney beans, chickpeas.
   - **Other Foods:** Cauliflower, asparagus, zucchini.

2. Yellow Foods
   - **Fruits:** Bananas, oranges, apples, pears.
   - **Whole Grains:** Brown rice, oats, quinoa, barley.
   - **Lean Proteins:** Chicken breast, salmon, tofu, lean beef.
   - **Starchy Vegetables:** Sweet potatoes, corn, butternut squash.
   - **Other Foods:** Low-fat dairy products, whole-grain pasta.

3. Red Foods
   - **Processed Snacks:** Chips, cookies, candy.
   - **Sugary Beverages:** Soda, fruit juices with added sugar.
   - **High-Fat Meats:** Bacon, sausage, fatty cuts of beef.
   - **Desserts:** Cakes, pastries, ice cream.
   - **Other Foods:** White bread, sugary cereals.

MENU TEMPLATES FOR BREAKFAST, LUNCH, DINNER AND SNACKS.

Sample Breakfast Menu
1. Green Smoothie Bowl
2. Avocado and Tomato Toast on Whole Grain Bread
3. Apple Cinnamon Overnight Oats
4. Greek Yogurt with Berries and Chia Seeds
5. Chia Seed Pudding with Berries

Sample Lunch Menu
1. Quinoa and Vegetable Salad
2. Stuffed Bell Peppers with Quinoa
3. Lentil and Spinach Stew
4. Sweet Potato and Black Bean Tacos
5. Grilled Vegetable and Hummus Wrap

Sample Dinner Menu
1. Grilled Lemon Herb Chicken
2. Salmon with Asparagus
3. Chicken and Broccoli Alfredo (with Zoodles)
4. Grilled Pork Tenderloin with Apples
5. Lemon Garlic Shrimp over Zoodles

Sample Snack Menu
1. Greek Yogurt with Berries
2. Apple Slices with Almond Butter
3. Carrot and Ginger Smoothie
4. Cucumber and Mint Yogurt Dip
5. Mixed Berries with Cottage Cheese

BREAKFAST

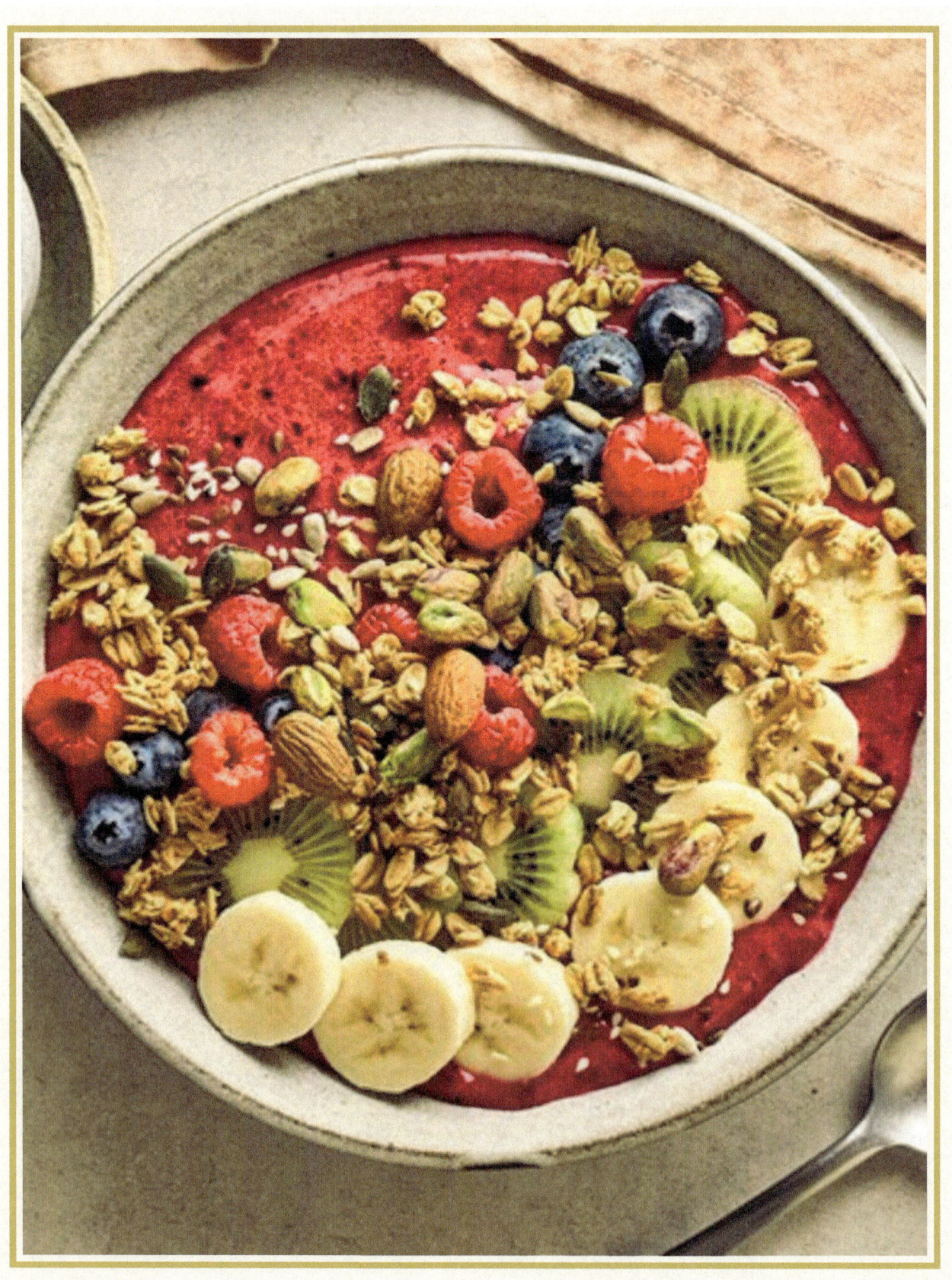

TABLE OF CONTENTS

- Green Smoothie Bowl (Green) — 14
- Spinach and Mushroom Omelette (Green) — 15
- Greek Yogurt with Berries and Chia Seeds (Green) — 16
- Mango and Spinach Smoothie (Green) — 17
- Tomato and Avocado Salad (Green) — 18
- Zoodle Salad with Lemon-Tahini Dressing (Green) — 19
- Apple Cinnamon Overnight Oats (Green) — 20
- Cucumber and Mint Yogurt Dip (Green) — 21
- Mixed Berries with Cottage Cheese (Green) — 22
- Kale and Sweet Potato Hash (Green) — 23
- Carrot and Ginger Smoothie (Green) — 24
- Quinoa Breakfast Bowl with Berries (Green) — 25
- Chia Seed Pudding with Berries (Green) — 26
- Tropical Green Smoothie (Green) — 27
- Pumpkin Spice Smoothie (Green) — 28
- Oatmeal with Flaxseed and Blueberries (Green) — 29
- Avocado Smoothie with Spinach (Green) — 30
- Blueberry Almond Overnight Oats (Green) — 31

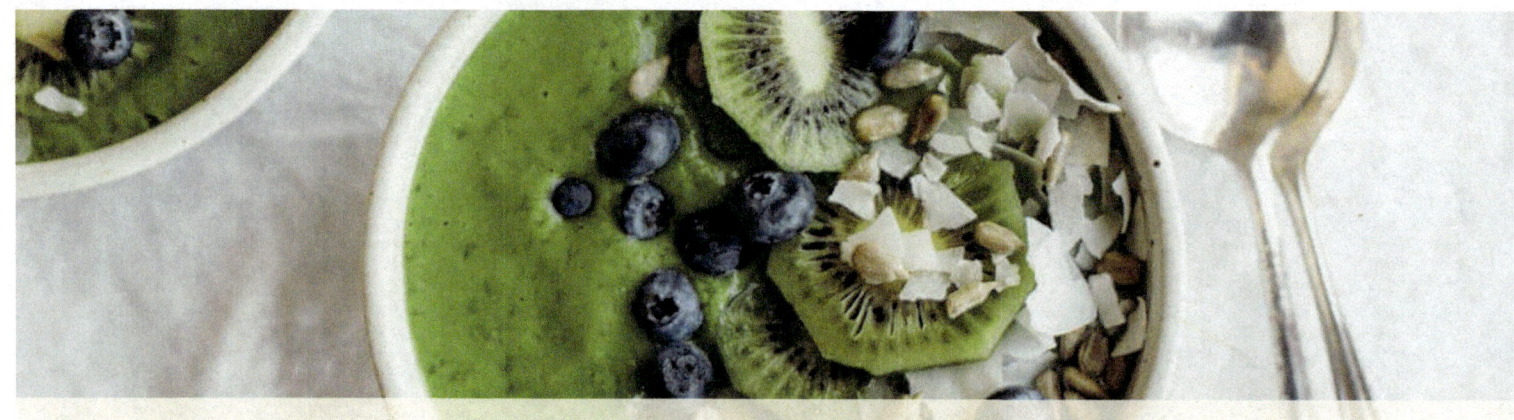

GREEN SMOOTHIE BOWL

The Green Smoothie Bowl is a nutritious and vibrant dish that combines leafy greens with wholesome ingredients, making it a perfect option for a balanced, Noom-friendly breakfast or snack. It's packed with vitamins, fiber, and healthy fats.

Serves	Preparation Time	Cooking Time 
4	5 minutes	4 minute

Ingredients:

1 cup fresh spinach or kale leaves
1/2 avocado
1/4 cup unsweetened almond milk (or coconut milk)
1/4 cup Greek yogurt (plain, low-fat)
1 tablespoon chia seeds
1 tablespoon almond butter or peanut butter (no sugar added)
1-2 tablespoons honey or maple syrup (optional, to taste)
Ice cubes (optional, for a thicker texture)

Toppings (optional):
Sliced almonds
Unsweetened shredded coconut
Fresh berries (like raspberries or blueberries)
Hemp seeds
Flaxseeds

Instructions:

1. **Blend the Smoothie:** In a blender, combine the spinach or kale, avocado, almond milk, Greek yogurt, chia seeds, almond butter, and sweetener (if using). Blend until smooth and creamy. If you prefer a thicker texture, add a few ice cubes and blend again.
2. **Assemble the Smoothie Bowl:** Pour the smoothie into a bowl. Add your favorite toppings such as sliced almonds, shredded coconut, fresh berries, hemp seeds, or flaxseeds.
3. **Serve:** Enjoy immediately as a refreshing and nourishing meal.

Nutrients (per serving)

Calories: 270 Sodium: 130 mg Carbohydrates: 14 g
Fiber: 7 g Protein: 9 g Calcium: 150 mg Fat: 21 g
Sugar: 5 g

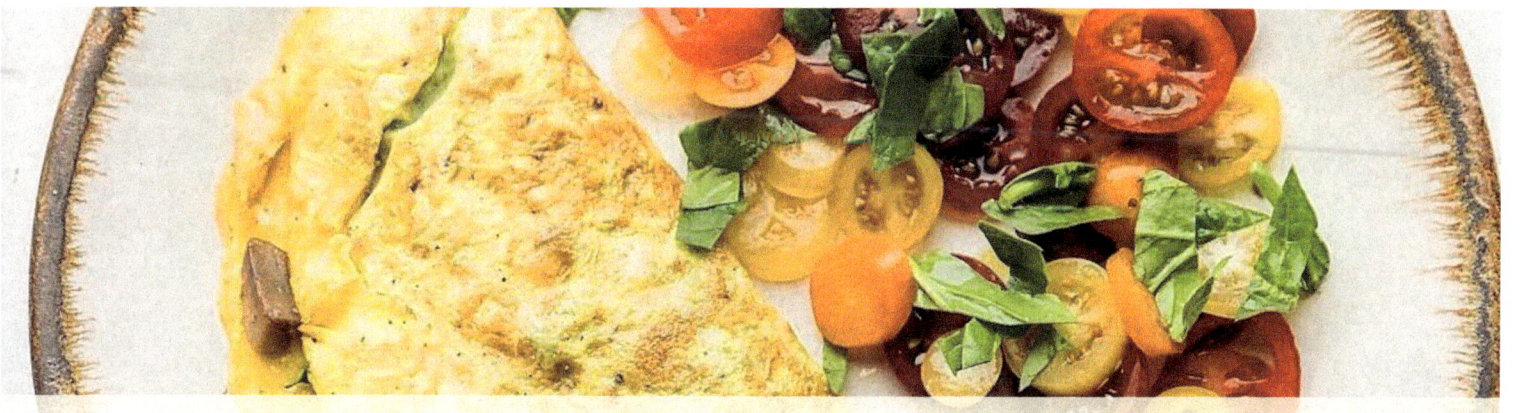

SPINACH AND MUSHROOM OMELETTE

The Spinach and Mushroom Omelette is a quick and nutritious meal, combining the earthy flavors of sautéed mushrooms with the freshness of spinach. It's perfect for a balanced breakfast or light lunch that aligns with your Noom goals.

Serves 	Preparation Time	Cooking Time
4	5 minutes	10 minute

Ingredients:

4 large eggs
1/2 cup fresh spinach leaves, chopped
1/2 cup mushrooms, sliced
1/4 cup onion, finely chopped
2 tablespoons milk (low-fat or plant-based)
1 tablespoon olive oil
Salt and pepper, to taste
Fresh parsley, chopped (optional, for garnish)

*Log as Spinach & Pea frittata. 166 C
1.25 servings 208 c
½ for 2.
Add cheese to Tom's.
feta for mine? add cals.*

Instructions:

1. **Prepare the Vegetables:** Heat olive oil in a non-stick skillet over medium heat. Add chopped onions and sauté until soft, about 2-3 minutes. Add sliced mushrooms and cook until they release their moisture and start to brown, about 4-5 minutes. Add spinach and cook until wilted, about 1-2 minutes. Season with salt and pepper. Remove the vegetables from the skillet and set aside.
2. **Cook the Omelette:** In a bowl, whisk together eggs, milk, salt, and pepper. Heat the same skillet over medium heat and add a little more oil if needed. Pour in the egg mixture, tilting the pan to spread it evenly. Cook for 2-3 minutes until the eggs start to set, then add the sautéed vegetables on one half of the omelette.
3. **Fold and Serve:** Gently fold the other half of the omelette over the vegetables. Continue cooking for another minute until the eggs are fully set. Slide the omelette onto a plate and garnish with fresh parsley if desired.

Nutrients (per serving)

Calories: 200 Sodium: 250 mg Carbohydrates: 5 g
Fiber: 1 g Protein: 15 g Calcium: 90 mg Fat: 14 g
Sugar: 2 g

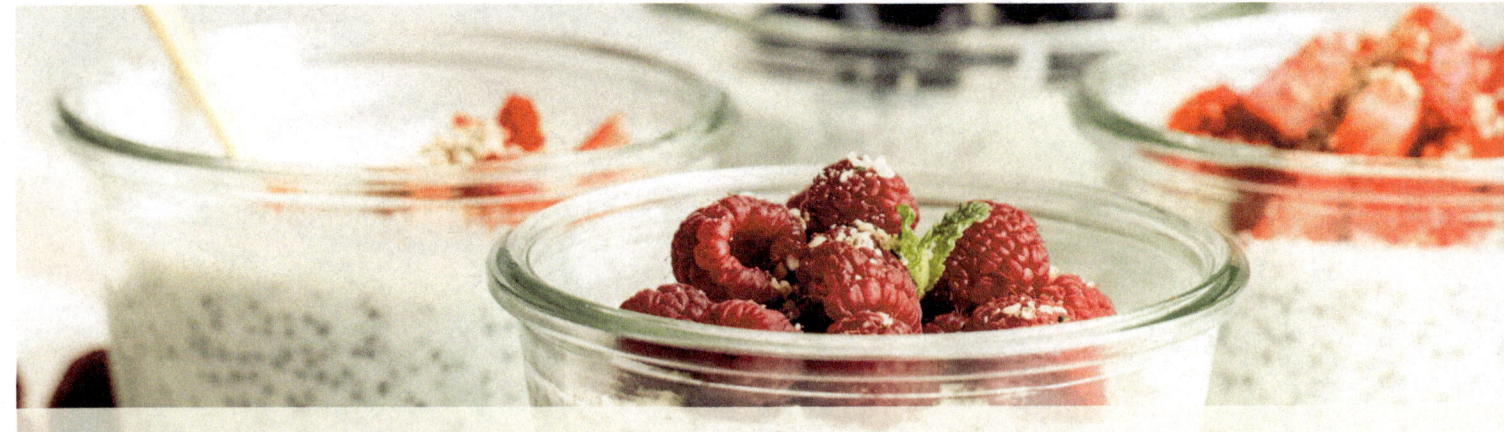

GREEK YOGURT WITH BERRIES AND CHIA SEEDS

Greek Yogurt with Berries and Chia Seeds is a simple yet satisfying dish, packed with protein, antioxidants, and fiber. It's an ideal breakfast or snack option for those following the Noom diet, providing a balanced mix of nutrients to keep you energized.

Serves: 4

Preparation Time: 5 minutes

Cooking Time: 0 minute

[handwritten: for 1.]

Ingredients:

- *[¼]* 1 cup plain Greek yogurt (low-fat or fat-free)
- *[⅛]* 1/2 cup mixed berries (strawberries, blueberries, raspberries)
- *[¼]* 1 tablespoon chia seeds
- *[¼]* 1 tablespoon honey or maple syrup (optional, to taste)
- *[drop]* 1/2 teaspoon vanilla extract (optional)

Instructions:

1. **Prepare the Yogurt:** In a bowl, mix the Greek yogurt with honey or maple syrup and vanilla extract if using. Stir until well combined.
2. **Assemble the Dish:** Spoon the yogurt into a serving bowl. Top with mixed berries and sprinkle with chia seeds.
3. **Serve:** Enjoy immediately as a refreshing and healthy breakfast or snack.

Nutrients (per serving)

Calories: 180 Sodium: 60 mg Carbohydrates: 24 g
Fiber: 5 g Protein: 13 g Calcium: 150 mg Fat: 5 g
Sugar: 15 g

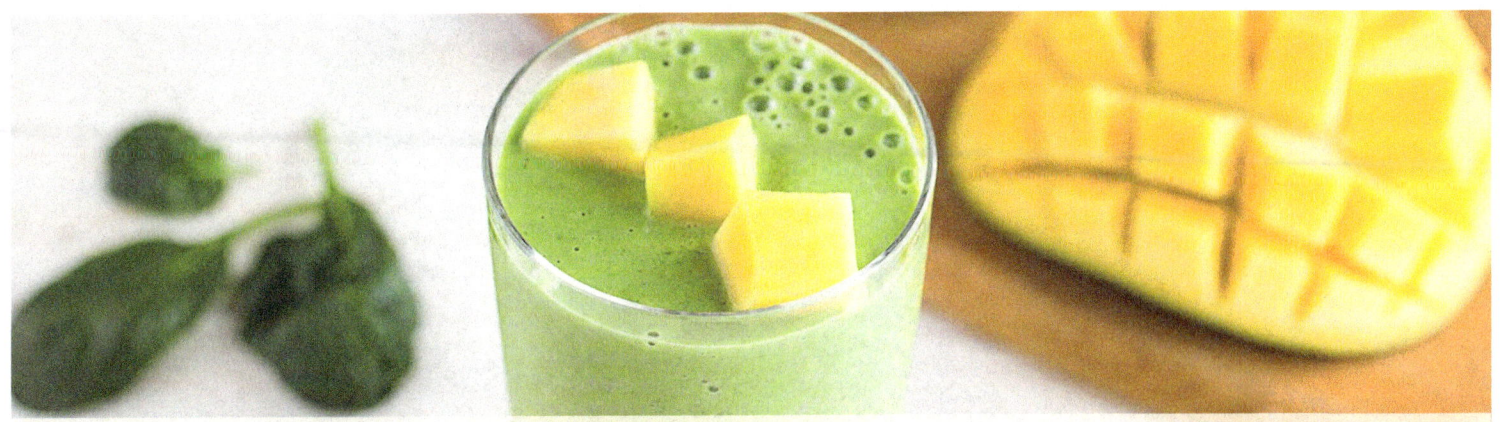

MANGO AND SPINACH SMOOTHIE

Mango and Spinach Smoothie is a refreshing and nutrient-packed drink, blending the sweetness of ripe mango with the vibrant greens of spinach. It's a perfect choice for a quick breakfast or a post-workout snack, providing essential vitamins and energy.

Serves 	Preparation Time	Cooking Time 
4	5 minutes	2 minute

②

Ingredients:

- 1 cup fresh or frozen mango chunks ½
- 1 cup fresh spinach leaves ½
- 1/2 banana (optional for added creaminess) ¼
- 1/2 cup Greek yogurt (plain, low-fat) ¼
- 1/2 cup unsweetened almond milk (or any milk of your choice) ¼
- 1 tablespoon chia seeds (optional) ½
- Ice cubes (optional, for a colder smoothie) ✓

Instructions:

1. **Prepare the Ingredients:** If using fresh mango, peel and cut the mango into chunks. Wash the spinach leaves thoroughly.
2. **Blend the Smoothie:** In a blender, combine the mango chunks, spinach leaves, banana (if using), Greek yogurt, almond milk, and chia seeds (if using).Blend until smooth and creamy. Add ice cubes if you prefer a colder smoothie and blend again until the ice is crushed.
3. **Serve:** Pour the smoothie into a glass and enjoy immediately.

Nutrients (per serving)

Calories: 210 Sodium: 70 mg Carbohydrates: 36 g

Fiber: 6 g Protein: 9 g Calcium: 150 mg Fat: 4 g

Sugar: 25 g

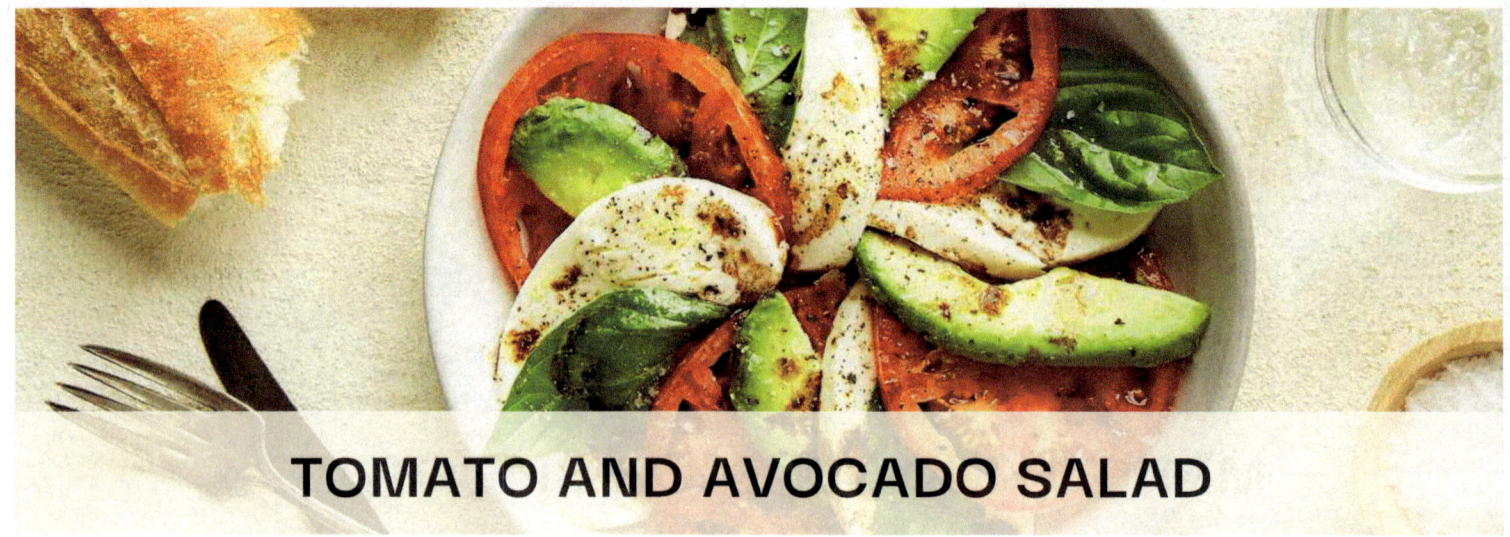

TOMATO AND AVOCADO SALAD

Tomato and Avocado Salad is a fresh and vibrant dish, combining juicy tomatoes with creamy avocado. It's a simple yet flavorful salad that makes a great side dish or light meal, aligning perfectly with a healthy eating plan.

Serves	Preparation Time	Cooking Time
4	10 minutes	0 minute

Ingredients:

- 2 ripe avocados, diced
- 2 large tomatoes, chopped
- 1/4 red onion, thinly sliced
- 1/4 cup fresh cilantro, chopped
- 1 tablespoon olive oil
- 1 tablespoon lemon or lime juice
- Salt and pepper, to taste
- Optional: 1/2 teaspoon cumin or chili flakes for extra flavor

(handwritten annotations in left margin: 1, 1, 1/8, 1/8, 1/2, 1/2, ✓, 1/4)
(handwritten annotations to the right: 1/2, 1/2, bit sliced, 1/4, 1/4, ✓)

Instructions:

1. **Prepare the Ingredients:** Dice the avocados and chop the tomatoes into bite-sized pieces. Thinly slice the red onion and chop the cilantro.
2. **Assemble the Salad:** In a large bowl, combine the diced avocado, chopped tomatoes, sliced red onion, and chopped cilantro. Drizzle with olive oil and lemon or lime juice. Add salt, pepper, and any additional seasonings to taste.
3. **Toss and Serve:** Gently toss the salad to ensure all ingredients are well mixed and evenly coated with the dressing. Serve immediately as a refreshing side dish or light meal.

Nutrients (per serving)

Calories: 200 Sodium: 150 mg Carbohydrates: 12 g
Fiber: 8 g Protein: 3 g Calcium: 20 mg Fat: 18 g
Sugar: 3 g

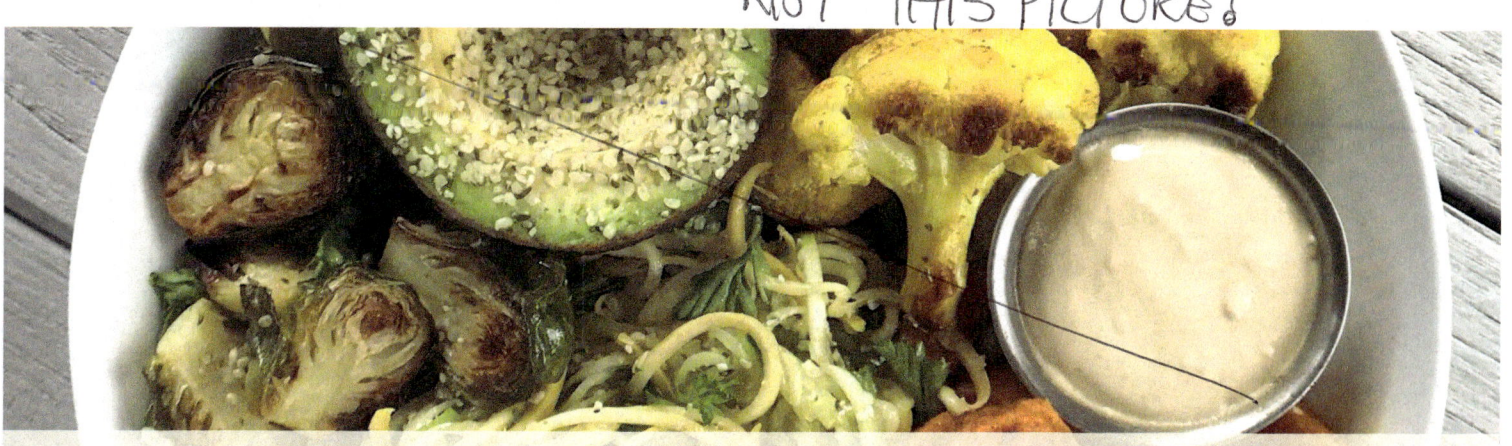

NOT THIS PICTURE!

ZOODLE SALAD WITH LEMON-TAHINI DRESSING

Zoodle Salad with Lemon-Tahini Dressing is a light and refreshing dish that replaces traditional pasta with zucchini noodles. Paired with a creamy, tangy dressing, it's a satisfying and healthy option for those looking to enjoy a fresh, nutrient-rich meal.

Serves	Preparation Time	Cooking Time
4	15 minutes	0 minute

Ingredients: ②

- 2 medium zucchinis, spiralized into zoodles 1
- 1 cup cherry tomatoes, halved 1/2
- 1/4 red onion, thinly sliced 1/8
- 1/4 cup fresh parsley, chopped 1/8
- 1/4 cup tahini 1/8
- 2 tablespoons lemon juice 1
- 1 tablespoon olive oil 1/2
- 1 clove garlic, minced —
- 1 tablespoon water (optional, to thin the dressing) 1/2
- Salt and pepper, to taste ✓
- Optional: 1/4 teaspoon ground cumin or smoked paprika for extra flavor 1/8

Instructions:

1. **Prepare the Zoodles:** Use a spiralizer to create zucchini noodles (zoodles). If you don't have a spiralizer, you can use a vegetable peeler to create thin zucchini strips.
2. **Prepare the Dressing:** In a small bowl, whisk together the tahini, lemon juice, olive oil, minced garlic, salt, pepper, and any optional seasonings. If the dressing is too thick, add water, one teaspoon at a time, until it reaches your desired consistency.
3. **Assemble the Salad:** In a large bowl, combine the zoodles, halved cherry tomatoes, sliced red onion, and chopped parsley. Drizzle the lemon-tahini dressing over the salad and toss gently to coat all the ingredients evenly.
4. **Serve:** Serve immediately as a refreshing and healthy salad.

Nutrients (per serving)

Calories: 150 Sodium: 120 mg Carbohydrates: 10 g
Fiber: 3 g Protein: 3 g Calcium: 30 mg Fat: 12 g
Sugar: 4 g

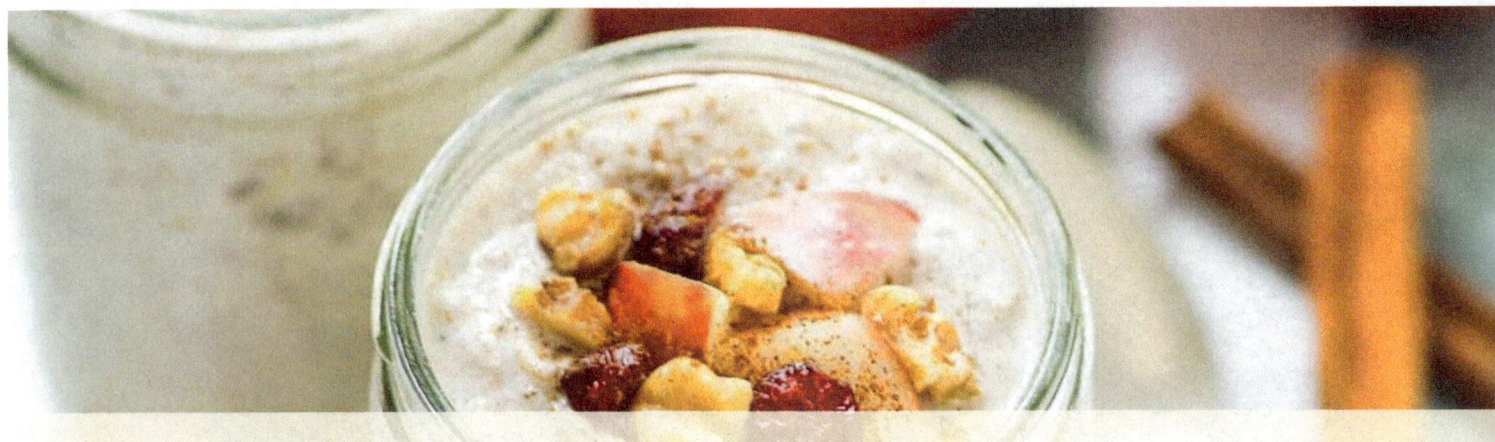

APPLE CINNAMON OVERNIGHT OATS

Apple Cinnamon Overnight Oats is a wholesome and convenient breakfast option that combines the comforting flavors of apples and cinnamon. Prepared the night before, this dish offers a quick and nutritious start to your day, packed with fiber and natural sweetness.

Serves	Preparation Time	Cooking Time
4 ✓	10 minutes	0 minute

Ingredients:

1 cup rolled oats
1 cup unsweetened almond milk (or any milk of your choice)
1/2 cup plain Greek yogurt
1 apple, diced
1 tablespoon chia seeds
1 tablespoon honey or maple syrup (optional)
1 teaspoon ground cinnamon
1/4 teaspoon vanilla extract
A pinch of salt
Optional toppings: chopped nuts, extra apple slices, or a sprinkle of cinnamon

Keep in fridge - 4 days.

Instructions:

1. **Combine Ingredients:** In a medium-sized bowl or jar, mix together the rolled oats, almond milk, Greek yogurt, chia seeds, honey or maple syrup (if using), ground cinnamon, vanilla extract, and salt. Stir in the diced apple until everything is well combined.
2. **Refrigerate Overnight:** Cover the bowl or jar with a lid or plastic wrap. Place in the refrigerator and let it sit overnight, or for at least 6 hours, to allow the oats to absorb the liquid and soften.
3. **Serve:** In the morning, give the oats a good stir. If the mixture is too thick, you can add a splash of almond milk to reach your desired consistency. Top with additional apple slices, chopped nuts, or a sprinkle of cinnamon before serving.

Nutrients (per serving)

Calories: 300 Sodium: 80 mg Carbohydrates: 50 g
Fiber: 8 g Protein: 10 g Calcium: 150 mg Fat: 6 g
Sugar: 15 g

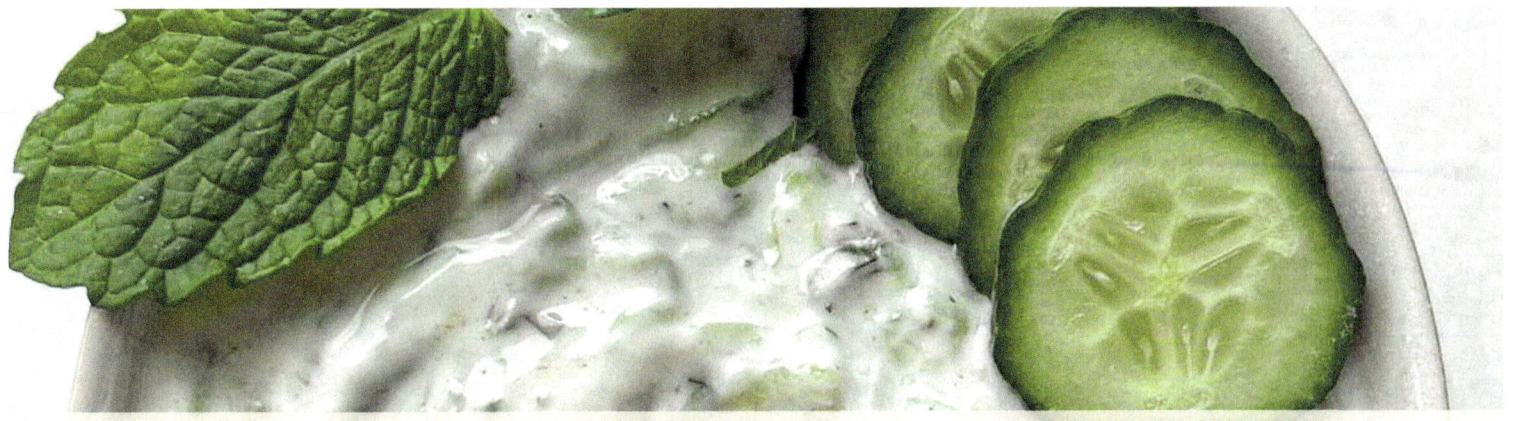

CUCUMBER AND MINT YOGURT DIP

Cucumber and Mint Yogurt Dip is a refreshing and light dip that combines creamy Greek yogurt with crisp cucumber and fresh mint. It's perfect as a snack or appetizer and pairs well with vegetables or whole-grain crackers.

"Tzatziki"

Serves	Preparation Time	Cooking Time
4	10 minutes	0 minute

Ingredients: ②

- 1 cup plain Greek yogurt (low-fat or fat-free) ½
- 1 medium cucumber, peeled, seeded, and finely diced ½
- 2 tablespoons fresh mint leaves, chopped 1
- 1 tablespoon lemon juice ½
- (1 clove garlic, minced)
- Salt and pepper, to taste
- Optional: 1 tablespoon olive oil for extra richness ½

Instructions:

1. **Prepare the Cucumber:** Peel the cucumber and remove the seeds using a spoon. Finely dice the cucumber.
2. **Mix the Dip:** In a bowl, combine the Greek yogurt, diced cucumber, chopped mint, lemon juice, and minced garlic. Stir well until all ingredients are evenly mixed.
3. **Season and Serve:** Add salt and pepper to taste. If using, stir in olive oil for a richer flavor. Chill the dip in the refrigerator for at least 30 minutes before serving to allow the flavors to meld. Serve with fresh vegetable sticks or whole-grain crackers.

Nutrients (per serving)

Calories: 80 Sodium: 40 mg Carbohydrates: 6 g

Fiber: 1 g Protein: 6 g Calcium: 80 mg Fat: 4 g

Sugar: 5 g

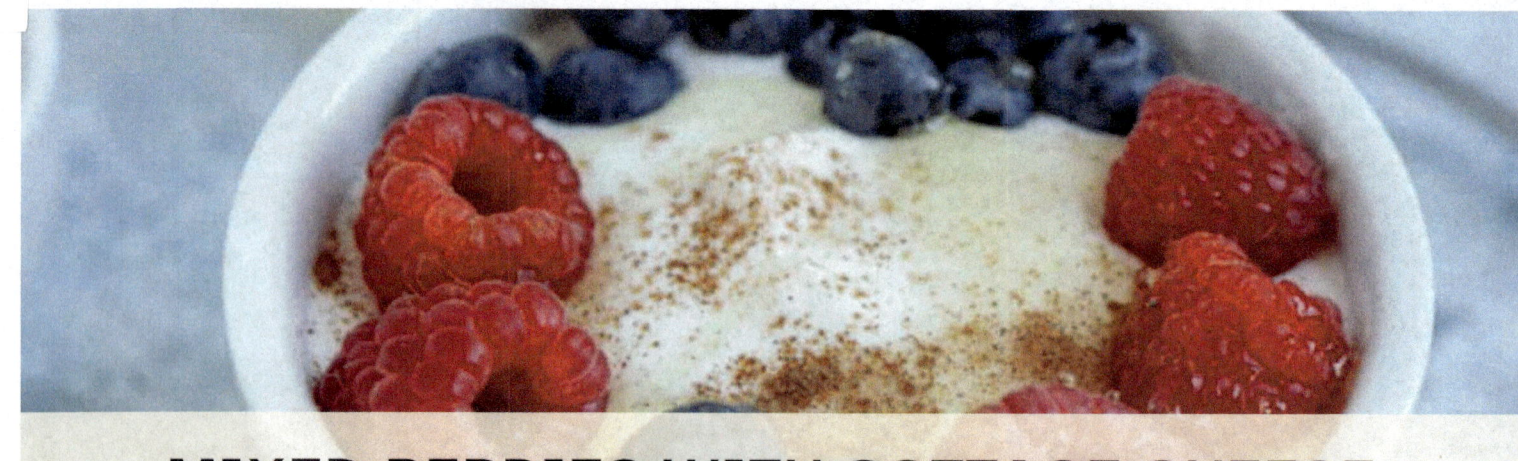

MIXED BERRIES WITH COTTAGE CHEESE

Mixed Berries with Cottage Cheese is a simple yet delicious dish that pairs the tartness of fresh berries with the creamy texture of cottage cheese. It's a nutritious and satisfying snack or light breakfast that offers a good balance of protein and antioxidants.

Serves	Preparation Time	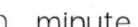 Cooking Time	
4	5 minutes	0 minute	

Ingredients:

- ¼ 1 cup mixed fresh berries (such as strawberries, blueberries, raspberries, and blackberries)
- ¼ 1 cup low-fat or fat-free cottage cheese
- ¼ 1 tablespoon honey or maple syrup (optional)
- ¼ 1 teaspoon lemon zest
- ¼ 1 tablespoon chopped nuts or seeds (optional, for added crunch)

Log as Bluberries + cheese 195c

¼ for 1

Not great.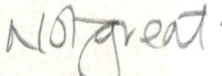

Instructions:

1. **Prepare the Berries:** Wash and pat dry the berries. If using large strawberries, slice them into smaller pieces.
2. **Mix with Cottage Cheese:** In a bowl, combine the cottage cheese and honey or maple syrup (if using). Stir to sweeten the cottage cheese to your taste.
3. **Assemble and Serve:** Spoon the sweetened cottage cheese into serving bowls. Top with mixed berries and a sprinkle of lemon zest. Add chopped nuts or seeds if desired for extra texture and crunch. Serve immediately.

Nutrients (per serving)

Calories: 180 Sodium: 400 mg Carbohydrates: 20 g
Fiber: 4 g Protein: 15 g Calcium: 200 mg Fat: 2 g
Sugar: 15 g

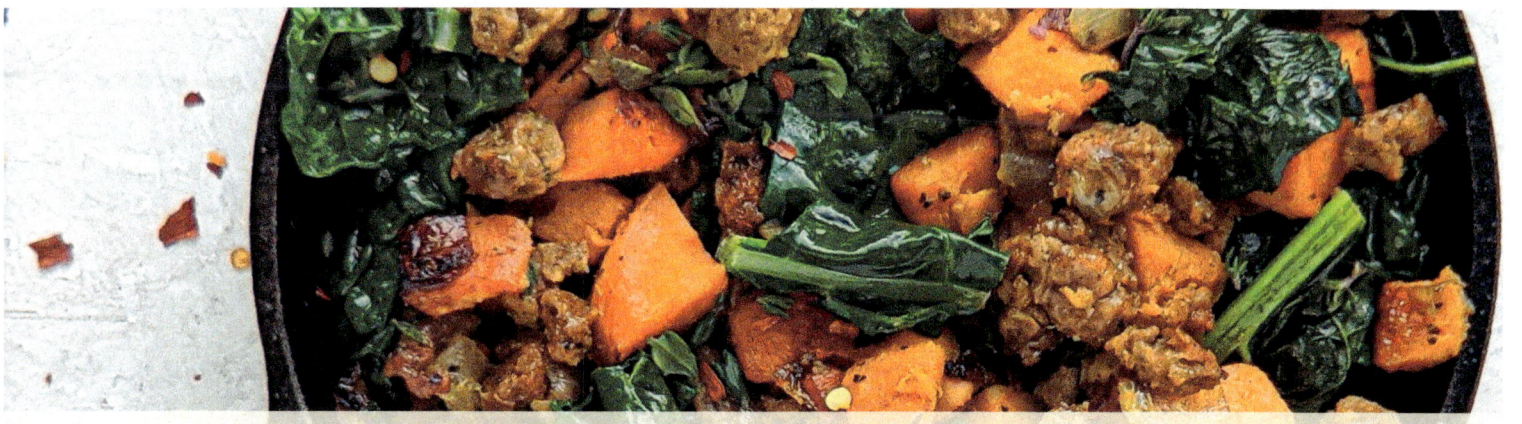

KALE AND SWEET POTATO HASH

Kale and Sweet Potato Hash is a hearty and nutritious dish that combines the earthy flavor of kale with the natural sweetness of roasted sweet potatoes. This versatile dish can be enjoyed for breakfast, lunch, or dinner, offering a delicious blend of textures and flavors.

Serves	Preparation Time	Cooking Time
4	10 minutes	30 minute

Ingredients: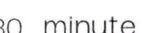

- 2 medium sweet potatoes, peeled and diced *(1)*
- 1 tablespoon olive oil *(½)*
- 1 small onion, diced *(½)*
- 2 cloves garlic, minced
- 2 cups fresh kale, chopped *(1)*
- 1/2 teaspoon paprika *(¼)*
- 1/2 teaspoon ground cumin *(¼)*
- Salt and pepper, to taste ✓
- Optional: 1/4 cup crumbled feta cheese or a sprinkle of red pepper flakes for extra flavor

Instructions:

1. **Prepare the Sweet Potatoes:** Preheat your oven to 400°F (200°C). Toss the diced sweet potatoes with half of the olive oil, salt, and pepper. Spread them out on a baking sheet and roast for 20-25 minutes, or until tender and slightly caramelized.
2. **Cook the Vegetables:** While the sweet potatoes are roasting, heat the remaining olive oil in a large skillet over medium heat. Add the diced onion and cook until softened and translucent, about 5 minutes. Add the minced garlic and cook for an additional 1-2 minutes, until fragrant.
3. **Add Kale and Spices:** Stir in the chopped kale and cook until wilted, about 3-4 minutes. Add paprika and ground cumin, and mix well.
4. **Combine and Serve:** Once the sweet potatoes are done, add them to the skillet with the kale mixture. Stir to combine and cook for an additional 2-3 minutes, allowing the flavors to meld. Adjust seasoning with salt and pepper, and sprinkle with crumbled feta cheese or red pepper flakes if desired.

Nutrients (per serving)

Calories: 220 Sodium: 150 mg Carbohydrates: 30 g
Fiber: 6 g Protein: 4 g Calcium: 80 mg Fat: 10 g
Sugar: 8 g

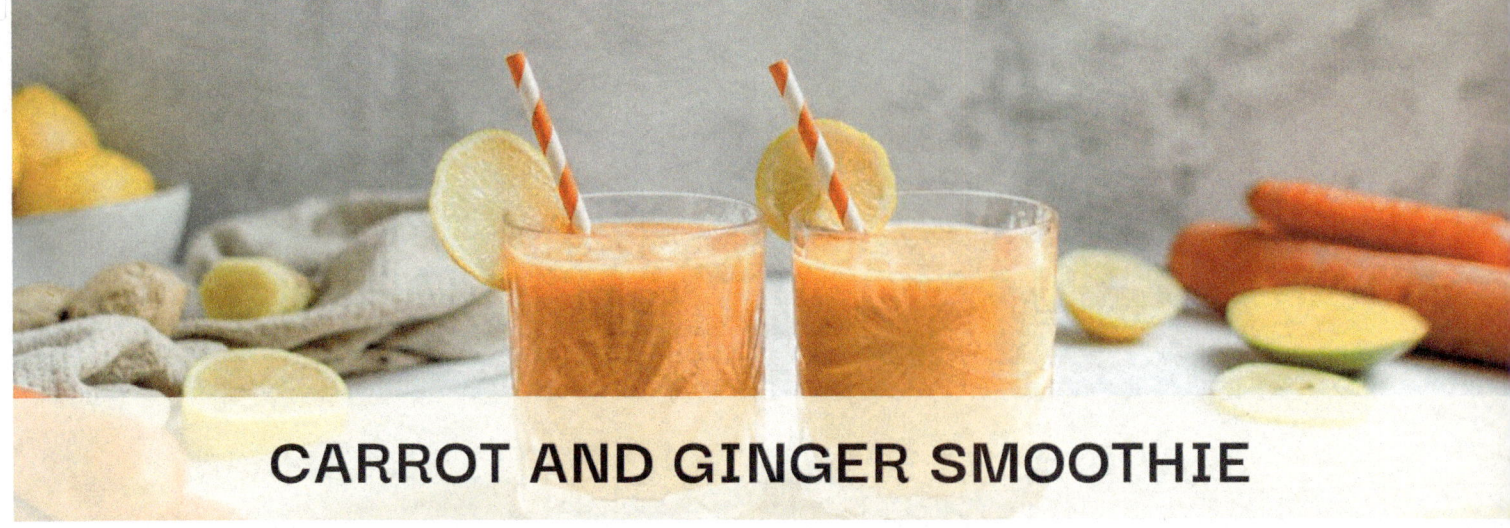

CARROT AND GINGER SMOOTHIE

Carrot and Ginger Smoothie is a refreshing and vibrant drink that combines the sweetness of carrots with the zing of fresh ginger. This nutrient-packed smoothie is rich in vitamins and antioxidants, making it a perfect choice for a healthy start to your day or a midday pick-me-up.

Serves	Preparation Time	Cooking Time	
4	10 minutes	0 minute	

Ingredients:

- 2 medium carrots, peeled and chopped
- 1 small piece of fresh ginger (about 1 inch), peeled and grated
- 1 cup orange juice (freshly squeezed if possible)
- 1/2 cup plain Greek yogurt
- 1 tablespoon honey or maple syrup (optional, for extra sweetness)
- 1/2 cup ice cubes
- Optional: 1/4 teaspoon ground turmeric for added health benefits

Instructions:

1. **Prepare the Ingredients:** Peel and chop the carrots. Peel and grate the ginger.
2. **Blend the Smoothie:** In a blender, combine the chopped carrots, grated ginger, orange juice, Greek yogurt, and honey or maple syrup (if using). Add ice cubes and blend until smooth. If the smoothie is too thick, add a bit more orange juice to reach your desired consistency.
3. **Serve:** Pour the smoothie into glasses and serve immediately. Optionally, sprinkle with ground turmeric for extra flavor and health benefits.

Nutrients (per serving)

Calories: 150 Sodium: 60 mg Carbohydrates: 35 g

Fiber: 4 g Protein: 6 g Calcium: 150 mg Fat: 1.5 g

Sugar: 25 g

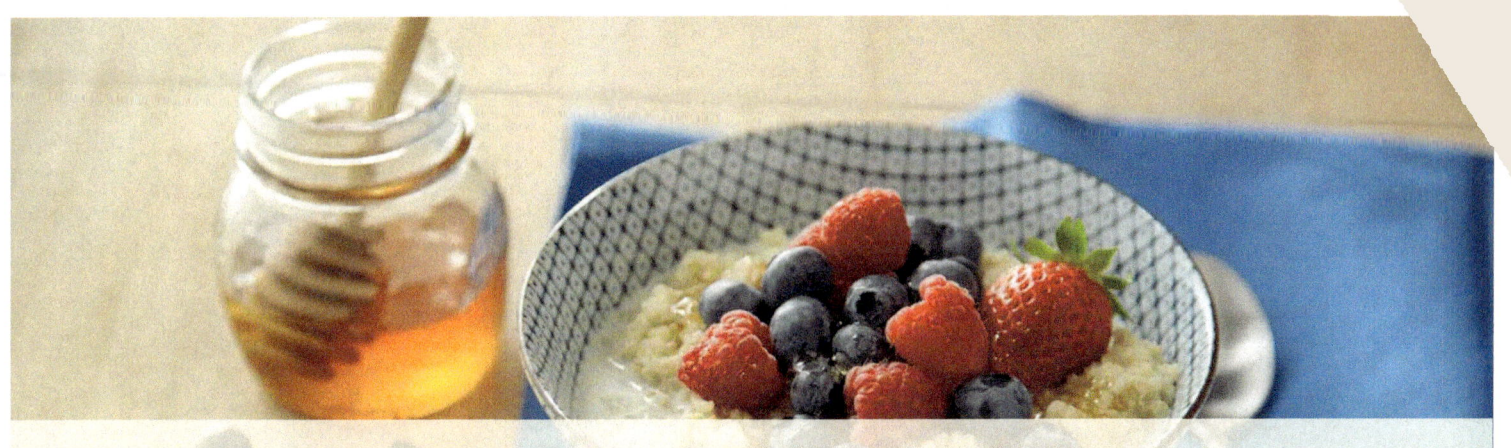

QUINOA BREAKFAST BOWL WITH BERRIES

Quinoa Breakfast Bowl with Berries is a wholesome and satisfying breakfast option that combines protein-packed quinoa with the fresh sweetness of mixed berries. This dish is not only nutritious but also customizable with various toppings and add-ins, making it a versatile choice for starting your day right.

Serves	Preparation Time	Cooking Time 
4	10 minutes	15 minute

Ingredients:

1 cup cooked quinoa (cooled)
1/2 cup mixed fresh berries (such as strawberries, blueberries, raspberries, and blackberries)
1/4 cup plain Greek yogurt
1 tablespoon honey or maple syrup (optional)
1 tablespoon chia seeds
1 tablespoon sliced almonds or walnuts (optional, for added crunch)
A sprinkle of cinnamon (optional)

Instructions:

1. **Prepare the Quinoa:** If you haven't already, cook 1/2 cup of dry quinoa according to package instructions. Allow it to cool before using.
2. **Assemble the Bowl:** In a serving bowl, place the cooked quinoa as the base. Top with fresh berries, Greek yogurt, and chia seeds. Drizzle with honey or maple syrup if you prefer extra sweetness.
3. **Add Optional Toppings:** Sprinkle with sliced almonds or walnuts for added crunch. Add a sprinkle of cinnamon for extra flavor if desired.
4. **Serve:** Serve immediately or refrigerate for a quick, grab-and-go breakfast option.

Nutrients (per serving)

Calories: 300 Sodium: 70 mg Carbohydrates: 40 g
Fiber: 6 g Protein: 12 g Calcium: 150 mg Fat: 8 g
Sugar: 15 g

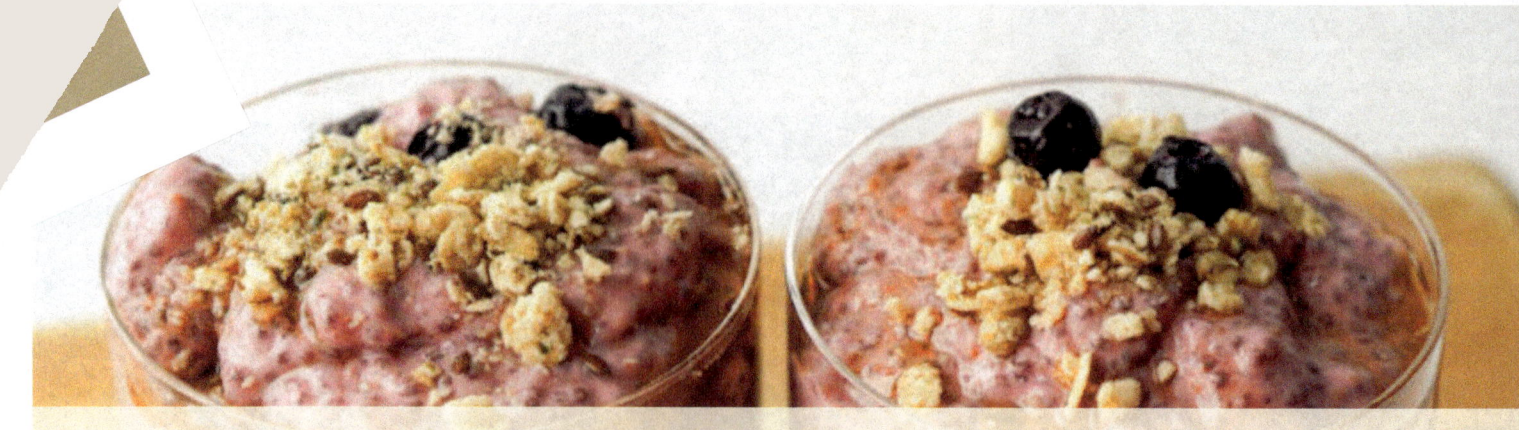

CHIA SEED PUDDING WITH BERRIES

Chia Seed Pudding with Berries is a creamy and nutritious breakfast or snack option that showcases the health benefits of chia seeds. Packed with fiber and omega-3 fatty acids, this delicious pudding is topped with fresh berries for a burst of flavor and antioxidants.

Serves	Preparation Time	Cooking Time	
4	10 minutes	0 minute	

Ingredients:

1/2 cup chia seeds
2 cups almond milk (or any milk of your choice)
2 tablespoons maple syrup or honey (optional, for sweetness)
1 teaspoon vanilla extract
1 cup mixed fresh berries (such as strawberries, blueberries, raspberries, and blackberries)
Optional toppings: sliced almonds, shredded coconut, or granola

Instructions:

1. **Prepare the Chia Pudding:** In a mixing bowl, combine chia seeds, almond milk, maple syrup or honey (if using), and vanilla extract. Stir well to ensure there are no clumps.
2. **Refrigerate:** Cover the bowl and refrigerate for at least 4 hours or overnight. The chia seeds will absorb the liquid and create a thick, pudding-like consistency.
3. **Serve:** Once the pudding has set, give it a good stir. Divide the pudding into serving bowls or glasses.
4. **Add Toppings:** Top each serving with fresh mixed berries and any optional toppings like sliced almonds, shredded coconut, or granola.
5. **Enjoy:** Serve immediately, or keep in the fridge for a quick and healthy breakfast or snack throughout the week.

Nutrients (per serving)

Calories: 180 Sodium: 25 mg Carbohydrates: 25 g
Fiber: 10 g Protein: 5 g Calcium: 150 mg Fat: 8 g
Sugar: 5 g

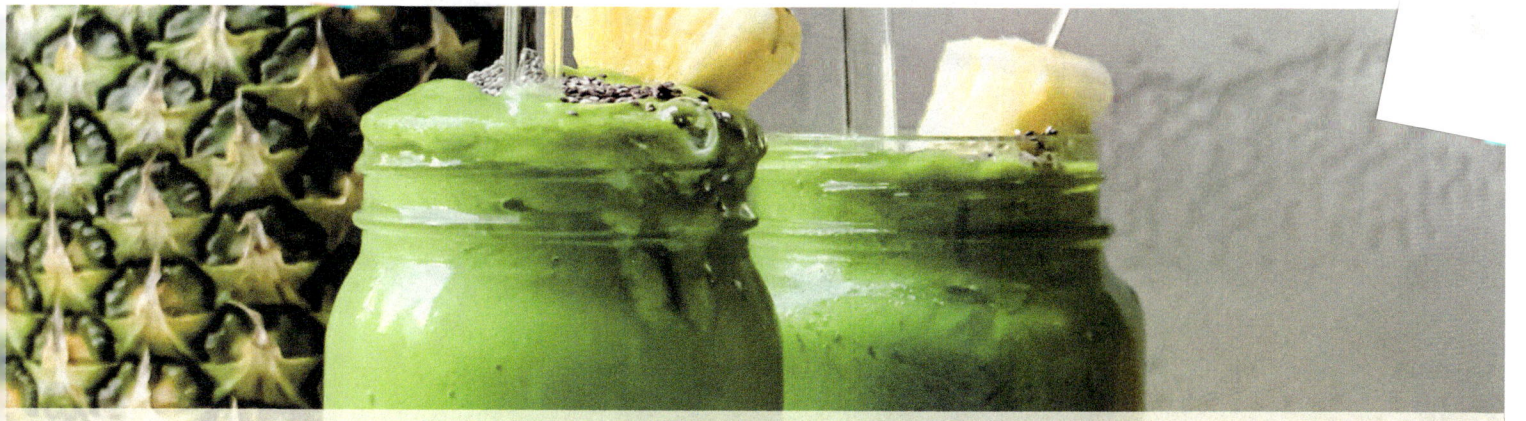

TROPICAL GREEN SMOOTHIE

Tropical Green Smoothie is a vibrant and refreshing drink that combines the goodness of leafy greens with the tropical flavors of pineapple and mango. This smoothie is packed with vitamins and minerals, making it a perfect choice for a nutritious start to your day or a revitalizing snack.

Serves		Preparation Time		Cooking Time	
4		5 minutes		0 minute	

Ingredients:

1 cup fresh spinach or kale leaves (stems removed)
1/2 cup frozen pineapple chunks
1/2 cup frozen mango chunks
1 banana, peeled
1 cup coconut water (or almond milk)
1 tablespoon chia seeds (optional, for added fiber and omega-3s)
1 teaspoon honey or maple syrup (optional, for extra sweetness)
A squeeze of lime juice (optional, for added tang)

Instructions:

1. **Prepare the Ingredients:** Wash and pat dry the spinach or kale. Peel the banana.
2. **Blend the Smoothie:** In a blender, combine the spinach or kale, frozen pineapple chunks, frozen mango chunks, banana, and coconut water. Add chia seeds and honey or maple syrup if using. Blend until smooth and creamy. If the smoothie is too thick, add a bit more coconut water to reach your desired consistency.
3. **Serve:** Pour the smoothie into glasses and serve immediately. Optionally, add a squeeze of lime juice for a zesty kick.

Nutrients (per serving)

Calories: 220 Sodium: 30 mg Carbohydrates: 50 g Fiber: 6 g Protein: 4 g Calcium: 60 mg Fat: 2 g Sugar: 30 g

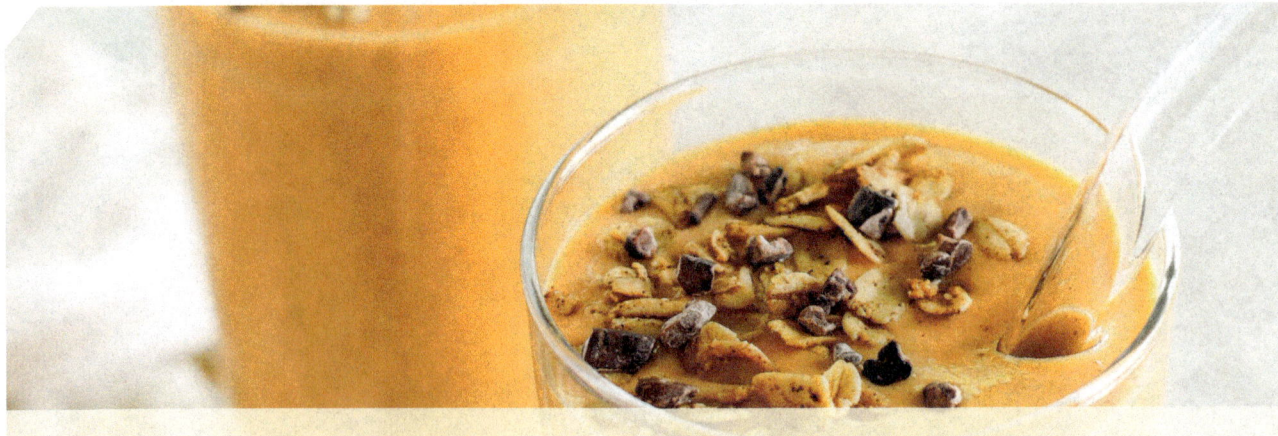

PUMPKIN SPICE SMOOTHIE

Pumpkin Spice Smoothie is a seasonal favorite that combines the rich, creamy texture of pumpkin with the warm, comforting spices of fall. Perfect for autumn, this smoothie is not only delicious but also packed with nutrients, making it a great choice for a healthy breakfast or a cozy snack.

Serves	Preparation Time	Cooking Time
4	5 minutes	0 minute

Ingredients:

1 cup canned pumpkin puree (not pumpkin pie filling)
1 banana, peeled
1/2 cup Greek yogurt (plain or vanilla)
1 cup almond milk (or any milk of your choice)
1 tablespoon maple syrup or honey (optional, for sweetness)
1/2 teaspoon pumpkin pie spice (or a mix of cinnamon, nutmeg, and cloves)
1/4 teaspoon vanilla extract
1/4 cup ice cubes

Instructions:

1. **Prepare the Ingredients:** Peel the banana.
2. **Blend the Smoothie:** In a blender, combine the pumpkin puree, banana, Greek yogurt, almond milk, maple syrup or honey (if using), pumpkin pie spice, and vanilla extract. Add ice cubes and blend until smooth and creamy. If the smoothie is too thick, add a bit more almond milk to reach your desired consistency.
3. **Serve:** Pour the smoothie into glasses and serve immediately. Optionally, sprinkle a pinch of pumpkin pie spice on top for extra flavor.

Nutrients (per serving)

Calories: 250 Sodium: 90 mg Carbohydrates: 35 g
Fiber: 6 g Protein: 10 g Calcium: 250 mg Fat: 6 g
Sugar: 20 g

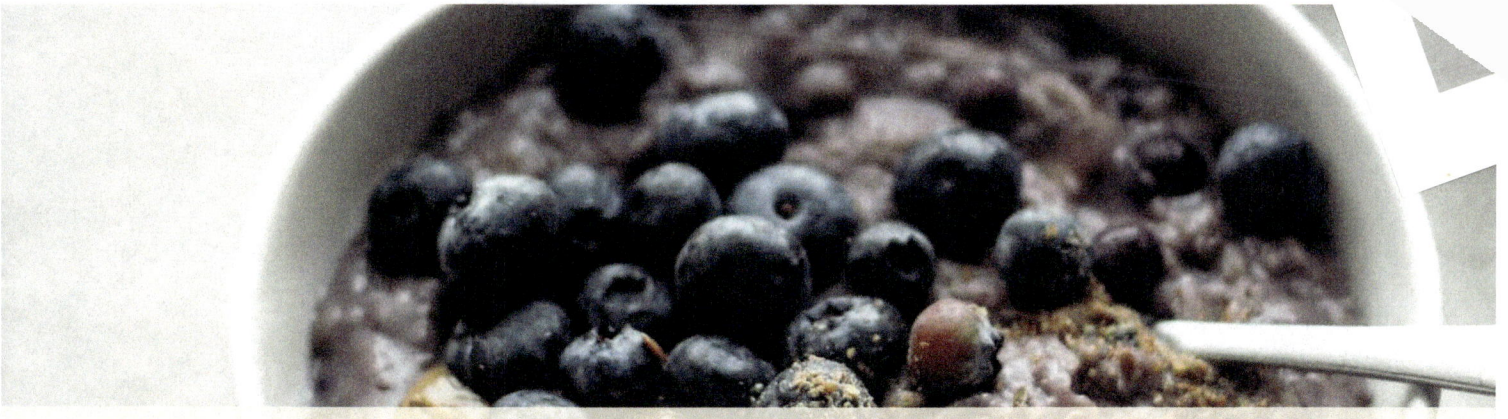

OATMEAL WITH FLAXSEED AND BLUEBERRIES

Oatmeal with Flaxseed and Blueberries is a wholesome and satisfying breakfast that combines the heartiness of oats with the nutritional benefits of flaxseeds and the antioxidant-rich sweetness of blueberries. This nutritious bowl provides a great start to your day, offering a balanced mix of fiber, healthy fats, and vitamins.

Serves	Preparation Time	Cooking Time
4	5 minutes	10 minute

Ingredients:

- 1 cup rolled oats — 1/4
- 2 cups water or almond milk (or any milk of your choice) — 1/2
- 1 tablespoon ground flaxseed — 1/4 1/8
- 1/2 cup fresh or frozen blueberries
- 1 tablespoon honey or maple syrup (optional, for sweetness) — 1/4
- 1/2 teaspoon vanilla extract (optional) ✓
- A pinch of salt ✓

Instructions:

1. **Cook the Oats:** In a medium saucepan, bring water or almond milk to a boil. Add the oats and a pinch of salt. Reduce heat to low and simmer, stirring occasionally, for 5-7 minutes, or until the oats are tender and the liquid is mostly absorbed.
2. **Add Flaxseed and Sweetener:** Stir in the ground flaxseed, honey or maple syrup (if using), and vanilla extract (if using). Cook for an additional 1-2 minutes, allowing the flavors to combine.
3. **Serve:** Spoon the oatmeal into bowls. Top with blueberries and any additional toppings you like, such as a sprinkle of flaxseed or a drizzle of honey.
4. **Enjoy:** Serve immediately and enjoy your warm, nourishing breakfast.

Nutrients (per serving)

Calories: 300 Sodium: 90 mg Carbohydrates: 50 g
Fiber: 8 g Protein: 8 g Calcium: 150 mg Fat: 8 g
Sugar: 12 g

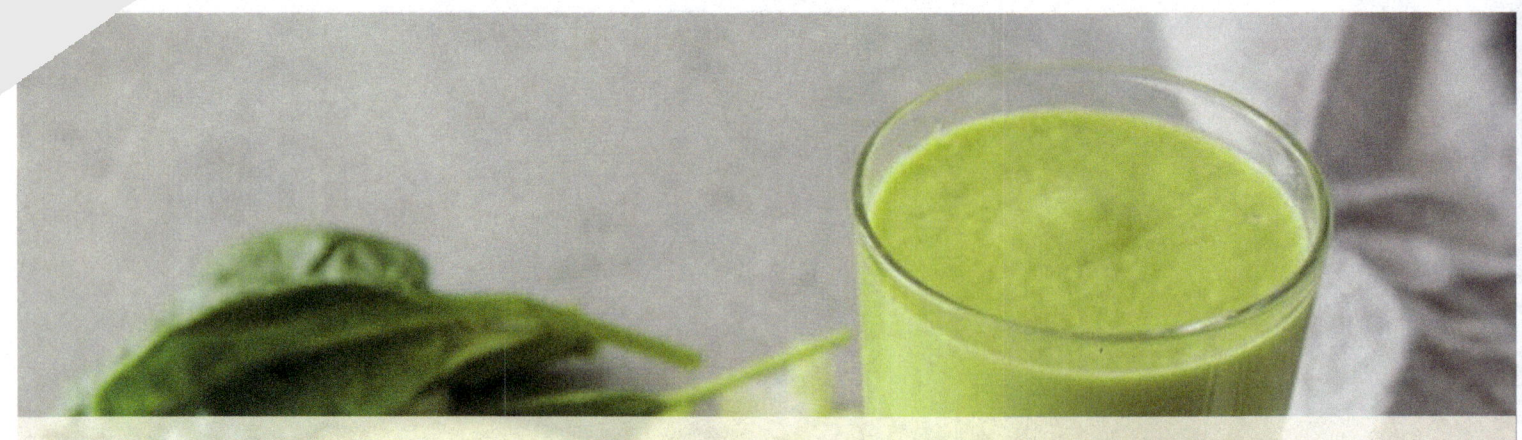

AVOCADO SMOOTHIE WITH SPINACH

Avocado Smoothie with Spinach is a creamy and nutritious drink that blends the rich, buttery flavor of avocado with the freshness of spinach. This smoothie is a powerhouse of vitamins and healthy fats, making it a great choice for a filling breakfast or a revitalizing snack.

Serves	Preparation Time	Cooking Time 
4	5 minutes	0 minute

Ingredients:

- 1 ripe avocado, peeled and pitted
- 1 cup fresh spinach leaves
- 1 banana, peeled
- 1 cup almond milk (or any milk of your choice)
- 1 tablespoon chia seeds (optional, for added fiber and omega-3s)
- 1 tablespoon honey or maple syrup (optional, for extra sweetness)
- 1/2 cup ice cubes
- A squeeze of lemon juice (optional, for added freshness)

Instructions:

1. **Prepare the Ingredients:** Peel and pit the avocado. Peel the banana.
2. **Blend the Smoothie:** In a blender, combine the avocado, spinach, banana, and almond milk. Add chia seeds and honey or maple syrup if using. Blend until smooth and creamy. If the smoothie is too thick, add a bit more almond milk to reach your desired consistency.
3. **Serve:** Pour the smoothie into glasses and serve immediately. Optionally, add a squeeze of lemon juice for a hint of freshness.

Nutrients (per serving)

Calories: 300 Sodium: 50 mg Carbohydrates: 40 g
Fiber: 10 g Protein: 6 g Calcium: 150 mg Fat: 15 g
Sugar: 15 g

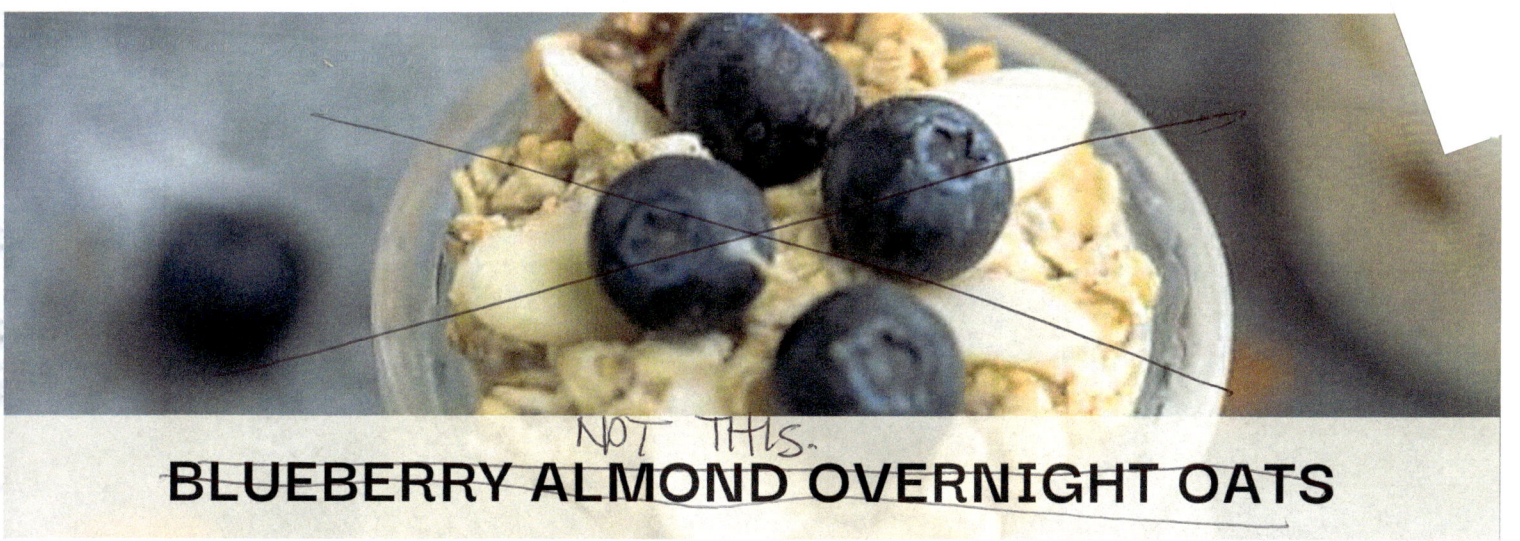

BLUEBERRY ALMOND OVERNIGHT OATS

NOT THIS.

Avocado Smoothie with Spinach is a creamy and nutritious drink that blends the rich, buttery flavor of avocado with the freshness of spinach. This smoothie is a powerhouse of vitamins and healthy fats, making it a great choice for a filling breakfast or a revitalizing snack.

AVOCADO SMOOTHIE

Serves	Preparation Time	Cooking Time
4	5 minutes	0 minute

Ingredients:

1 ripe avocado, peeled and pitted
1 cup fresh spinach leaves
1 banana, peeled
1 cup almond milk (or any milk of your choice)
1 tablespoon chia seeds (optional, for added fiber and omega-3s)
1 tablespoon honey or maple syrup (optional, for extra sweetness)
1/2 cup ice cubes
A squeeze of lemon juice (optional, for added freshness)

← *same recipe.*

Instructions:

1. **Prepare the Ingredients:** Peel and pit the avocado. Peel the banana.
2. **Blend the Smoothie:** In a blender, combine the avocado, spinach, banana, and almond milk. Add chia seeds and honey or maple syrup if using. Blend until smooth and creamy. If the smoothie is too thick, add a bit more almond milk to reach your desired consistency.
3. **Serve:** Pour the smoothie into glasses and serve immediately. Optionally, add a squeeze of lemon juice for a hint of freshness.

Nutrients (per serving)

Calories: 300 Sodium: 50 mg Carbohydrates: 40 g
Fiber: 10 g Protein: 6 g Calcium: 150 mg Fat: 15 g
Sugar: 15 g

LUNCH

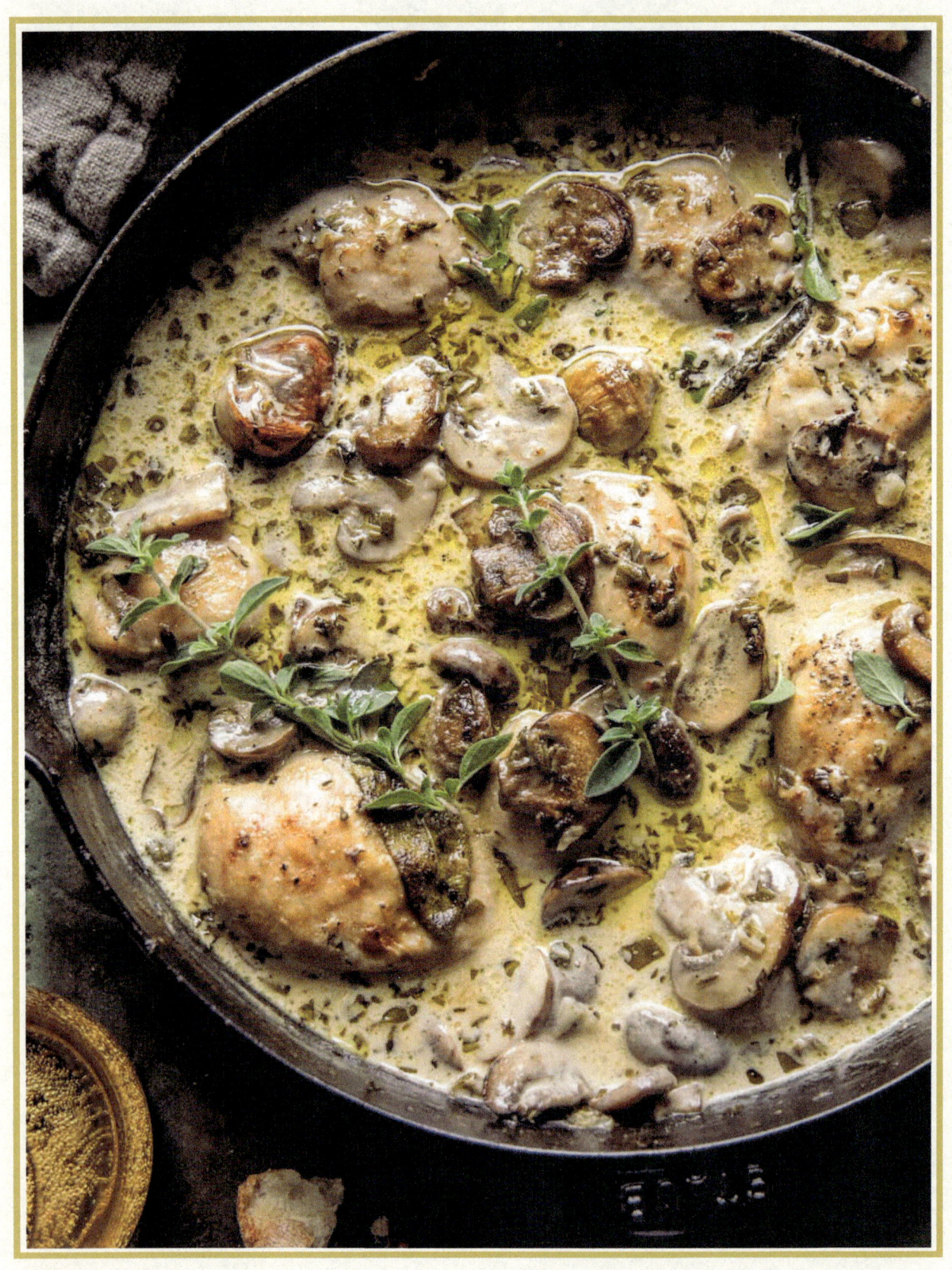

TABLE OF CONTENTS

- Quinoa and Vegetable Salad (Green) — 34
- Stuffed Bell Peppers with Quinoa (Green) — 35
- Cauliflower Rice Stir-Fry (Green) — 36
- Cucumber and Tomato Salad (Green) — 37
- Lentil and Spinach Stew (Green) — 38
- Kale and Apple Salad (Green) — 39
- Sweet Potato and Black Bean Tacos (Green) — 40
- Grilled Vegetable and Hummus Wrap (Green) — 41
- Broccoli and Cauliflower Soup (Green) — 42
- Tomato and Cucumber Quinoa Salad (Green) — 43
- Chickpea and Avocado Salad (Green) — 44
- Spinach and Feta Stuffed Mushrooms (Green) — 45
- Roasted Beet and Goat Cheese Salad (Green) — 46
- Sweet Potato and Chickpea Curry (Green) — 47
- Mediterranean Zoodle Salad (Green) — 48
- Roasted Butternut Squash Soup (Green) — 49
- Vegetable and Lentil Soup (Green) — 50
- Grilled Asparagus and Quinoa Salad (Green) — 51

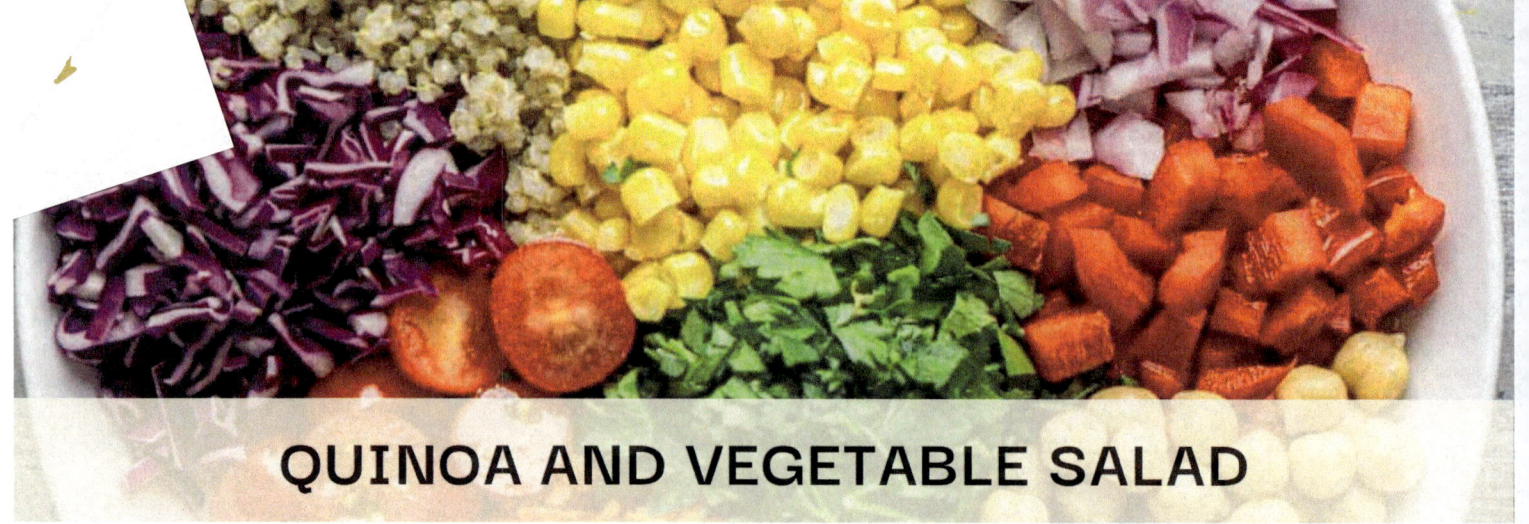

QUINOA AND VEGETABLE SALAD

Quinoa and Vegetable Salad is a vibrant, nutrient-rich dish that combines the nutty flavor of quinoa with a variety of fresh vegetables. This salad is light yet filling, making it a perfect option for a healthy lunch or side dish. Packed with fiber, protein, and vitamins, it supports overall wellness and energy.

Serves	Preparation Time	Cooking Time
4	10 minutes	15 minute

Ingredients:

1 cup quinoa, rinsed
2 cups water or vegetable broth
1 cup cherry tomatoes, halved
1 cucumber, diced
1 red bell pepper, diced
1/2 red onion, finely chopped
1/4 cup fresh parsley or cilantro, chopped
1/4 cup crumbled feta cheese (optional)
2 tablespoons olive oil
1 tablespoon lemon juice
1 teaspoon Dijon mustard
Salt and pepper to taste

Instructions:

1. **Cook the Quinoa:** In a medium saucepan, bring water or vegetable broth to a boil. Add the rinsed quinoa, reduce heat to low, cover, and simmer for 15 minutes, or until the quinoa is tender and the liquid is absorbed. Remove from heat and let it cool.
2. **Prepare the Vegetables:** While the quinoa is cooling, chop the cherry tomatoes, cucumber, red bell pepper, and red onion. Set aside.
3. **Make the Dressing:** In a small bowl, whisk together the olive oil, lemon juice, Dijon mustard, salt, and pepper.
4. **Assemble the Salad:** In a large bowl, combine the cooked quinoa with the chopped vegetables and fresh herbs. Drizzle with the dressing and toss to coat evenly.
5. **Serve:** Top with crumbled feta cheese, if using, and serve the salad chilled or at room temperature.

Lunch.
Supper w- fish/chicken

Nutrients (per serving)

Calories: 210 Sodium: 75 mg Carbohydrates: 30 g
Fiber: 5 g Protein: 6 g Calcium: 60 mg Fat: 8 g
Sugar: 4 g

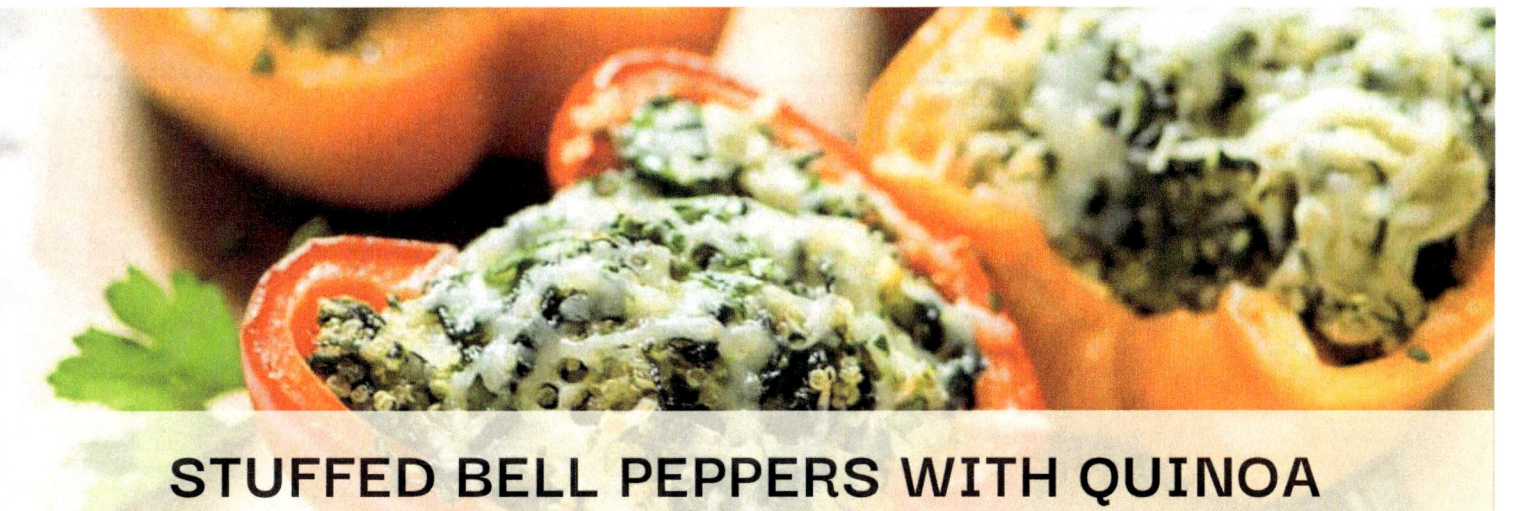

STUFFED BELL PEPPERS WITH QUINOA

Stuffed Bell Peppers with Quinoa is a hearty and colorful dish that combines the wholesome goodness of quinoa with savory vegetables, all packed into sweet bell peppers. This dish is not only visually appealing but also rich in protein, fiber, and essential nutrients, making it a satisfying and nutritious meal.

Serves	Preparation Time	Cooking Time
4	15 minutes	45 minute

Ingredients:

- 4 large bell peppers (any color)
- 1 cup quinoa, rinsed
- 2 cups vegetable broth or water
- 1 small onion, finely chopped
- 1 zucchini, diced
- 1 cup cherry tomatoes, halved
- 1 cup canned black beans, drained and rinsed
- 1 teaspoon cumin
- 1 teaspoon smoked paprika
- 1/2 teaspoon garlic powder
- 1/2 teaspoon salt
- 1/4 teaspoon black pepper
- 1/4 cup fresh cilantro, chopped
- 1/2 cup shredded cheese (optional)
- 1 tablespoon olive oil

Instructions:

1. **Cook the Quinoa:** In a medium saucepan, bring the vegetable broth or water to a boil. Add the rinsed quinoa, reduce heat to low, cover, and simmer for 15 minutes, or until the quinoa is tender and the liquid is absorbed. Fluff with a fork and set aside.
2. **Prepare the Bell Peppers:** Preheat the oven to 375°F (190°C). Slice the tops off the bell peppers and remove the seeds and membranes. Lightly brush the outside of the peppers with olive oil and place them in a baking dish.
3. **Cook the Filling:** In a large skillet, heat olive oil over medium heat. Add the chopped onion and sauté until softened, about 3-4 minutes. Add the diced zucchini and cherry tomatoes, and cook for another 5 minutes until the vegetables are tender. Stir in the cooked quinoa, black beans, cumin, smoked paprika, garlic powder, salt, and black pepper. Mix well to combine. Remove from heat and stir in the fresh cilantro.
4. **Stuff the Peppers:** Spoon the quinoa and vegetable mixture into each bell pepper, packing it tightly. If using, sprinkle the top with shredded cheese.
5. **Bake:** Cover the baking dish with foil and bake for 25 minutes. Remove the foil and bake for an additional 10 minutes, or until the peppers are tender and the cheese is melted and bubbly.
6. **Serve:** Allow the stuffed peppers to cool slightly before serving. Garnish with extra cilantro if desired.

Nutrients (per serving)

Calories: 300 Sodium: 350 mg Carbohydrates: 45 g
Fiber: 10 g Protein: 10 g Calcium: 100 mg Fat: 9 g
Sugar: 8 g

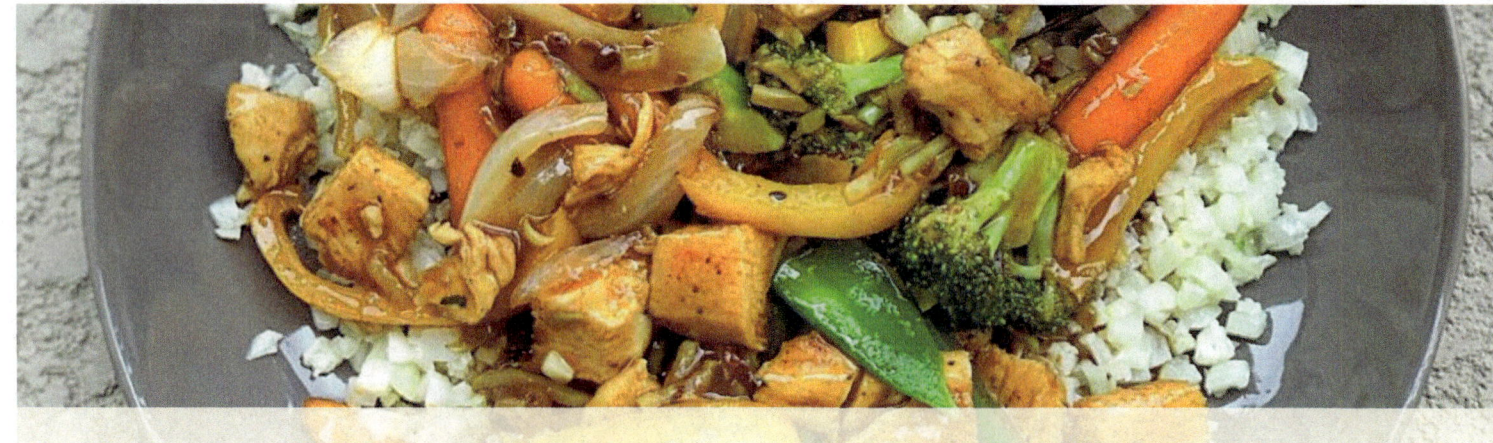

CAULIFLOWER RICE STIR-FRY

Cauliflower Rice Stir-Fry is a light, flavorful, and low-carb alternative to traditional fried rice. This dish features finely chopped cauliflower as a substitute for rice, combined with fresh vegetables and seasonings for a nutritious and satisfying meal.

Serves	Preparation Time 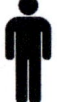	Cooking Time 
4	10 minutes	15 minute

Ingredients:

1 medium head of cauliflower, grated or processed into rice-sized pieces
1 tablespoon olive oil
1 small onion, finely chopped
2 cloves garlic, minced
1 cup carrots, diced
1 cup bell peppers, diced
1 cup snap peas or green beans, chopped
2 eggs, lightly beaten
3 tablespoons soy sauce or tamari (for gluten-free)
1 tablespoon sesame oil
1/2 teaspoon ground ginger
1/4 teaspoon black pepper
2 green onions, sliced (for garnish)
1 tablespoon sesame seeds (optional

Scramble eggs separately, add at step 5. w. some cooked prawns / cooked chicken

Instructions:

1. **Prepare the Cauliflower Rice:** Grate the cauliflower using a box grater or pulse in a food processor until it resembles rice. Set aside.
2. **Cook the Vegetables:** Heat the olive oil in a large skillet or wok over medium heat. Add the chopped onion and garlic, and sauté until softened and fragrant, about 3-4 minutes. Add the diced carrots, bell peppers, and snap peas (or green beans) to the skillet. Cook, stirring occasionally, for 5-7 minutes, until the vegetables are tender but still crisp.
3. **Cook the Eggs:** Push the vegetables to one side of the skillet and pour the beaten eggs into the empty space. Scramble the eggs until fully cooked, then mix them with the vegetables.
4. **Add the Cauliflower Rice:** Add the cauliflower rice to the skillet, stirring to combine with the vegetables and eggs. Cook for 5-7 minutes, until the cauliflower rice is tender and heated through.
5. **Season the Stir-Fry:** Stir in the soy sauce, sesame oil, ground ginger, and black pepper. Mix well to evenly coat the cauliflower rice and vegetables with the seasoning.
6. **Serve:** Garnish with sliced green onions and sesame seeds, if desired. Serve hot as a main dish or side.

Nutrients (per serving)

Calories: 150 Sodium: 500 mg Carbohydrates: 15 g
Fiber: 5 g Protein: 7 g Calcium: 40 mg Fat: 8 g
Sugar: 5 g

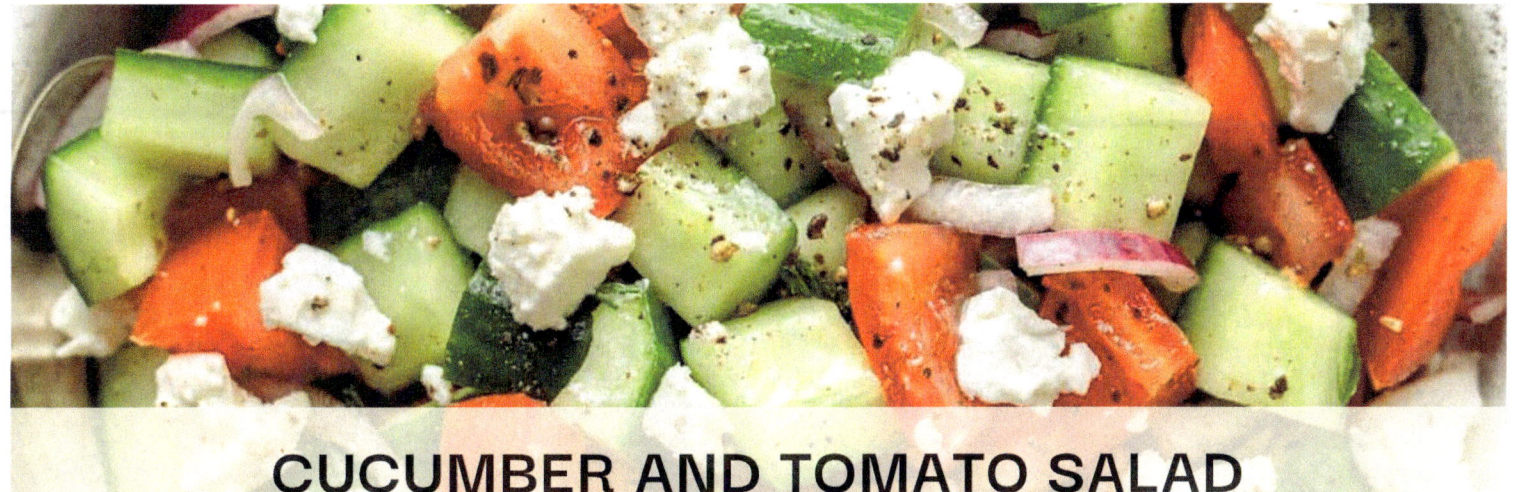

CUCUMBER AND TOMATO SALAD

Cucumber and Tomato Salad is a refreshing and simple dish that highlights the natural flavors of fresh vegetables. It's perfect as a light side dish or a healthy snack, offering a crisp and juicy combination that's both satisfying and nutritious.

Serves
4

Preparation Time
10 minutes

Cooking Time
0 minute

Ingredients:

2 large cucumbers, sliced
3 medium tomatoes, chopped
1/2 red onion, thinly sliced
2 tablespoons olive oil
1 tablespoon ~~red wine vinegar~~ or lemon juice
1 teaspoon dried oregano or basil
Salt and black pepper to taste
Fresh parsley or cilantro, chopped (for garnish)

+ feta!

Instructions:

1. **Prepare the Vegetables:** In a large bowl, combine the sliced cucumbers, chopped tomatoes, and thinly sliced red onion.
2. **Make the Dressing:** In a small bowl, whisk together the olive oil, red wine vinegar (or lemon juice), dried oregano (or basil), salt, and black pepper.
3. **Toss the Salad:** Pour the dressing over the cucumber and tomato mixture. Toss gently to ensure the vegetables are evenly coated with the dressing.
4. **Serve:** Garnish with chopped fresh parsley or cilantro. Serve immediately, or chill in the refrigerator for 10-15 minutes before serving for an extra refreshing taste.

Nutrients (per serving)

Calories: 80 Sodium: 150 mg Carbohydrates: 7 g
Fiber: 2 g Protein: 1 g Calcium: 20 mg Fat: 6 g
Sugar: 4 g

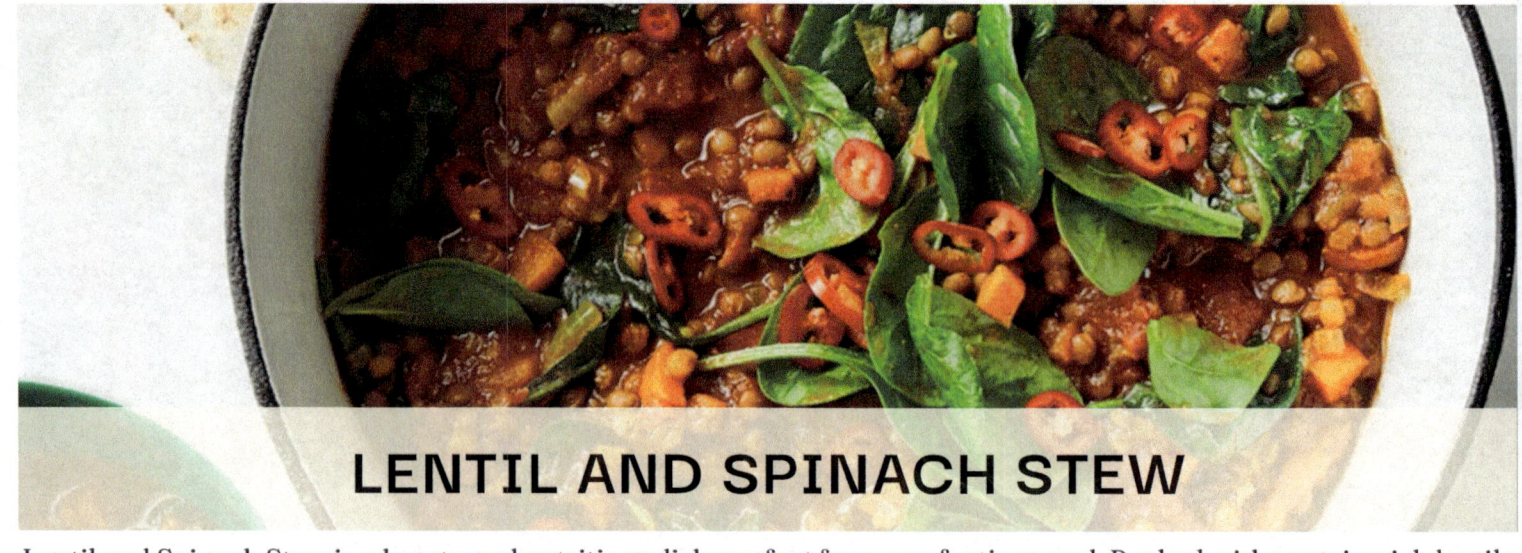

LENTIL AND SPINACH STEW

Lentil and Spinach Stew is a hearty and nutritious dish, perfect for a comforting meal. Packed with protein-rich lentils and nutrient-dense spinach, this stew is both satisfying and flavorful, making it an ideal option for a wholesome lunch or dinner.

Serves 	Preparation Time 	Cooking Time 
4	10 minutes	40 minute

Ingredients:

1 cup dried lentils, rinsed and drained
1 tablespoon olive oil
1 medium onion, chopped
2 cloves garlic, minced
2 carrots, diced
2 celery stalks, diced
1 can (14.5 oz) diced tomatoes, with juice
4 cups vegetable broth or water
1 teaspoon ground cumin
1/2 teaspoon ground coriander
1/2 teaspoon paprika
Salt and black pepper to taste
4 cups fresh spinach, chopped
Juice of 1 lemon (optional)
Fresh parsley, chopped (for garnish)

Instructions:

1. **Sauté the Aromatics:** Heat olive oil in a large pot over medium heat. Add the chopped onion and garlic, sautéing until the onion is translucent and fragrant, about 3-4 minutes.
2. **Add the Vegetables:** Stir in the diced carrots and celery, cooking for another 5 minutes until the vegetables begin to soften.
3. **Cook the Lentils:** Add the lentils, diced tomatoes (with juice), vegetable broth, ground cumin, coriander, paprika, salt, and black pepper to the pot. Stir well to combine.
4. **Simmer the Stew:** Bring the mixture to a boil, then reduce the heat to low. Cover the pot and let it simmer for 25-30 minutes, or until the lentils are tender and the flavors have melded together.
5. **Add the Spinach:** Stir in the chopped spinach and cook for an additional 5 minutes, until the spinach is wilted. If desired, add the lemon juice for a bright, tangy finish.
6. **Serve:** Ladle the stew into bowls and garnish with chopped fresh parsley. Serve hot, with crusty bread or over rice for a more filling meal.

Nutrients (per serving)

Calories: 220 Sodium: 350 mg Carbohydrates: 32 g
Fiber: 11 g Protein: 12 g Calcium: 100 mg Fat: 4 g
Sugar: 7 g

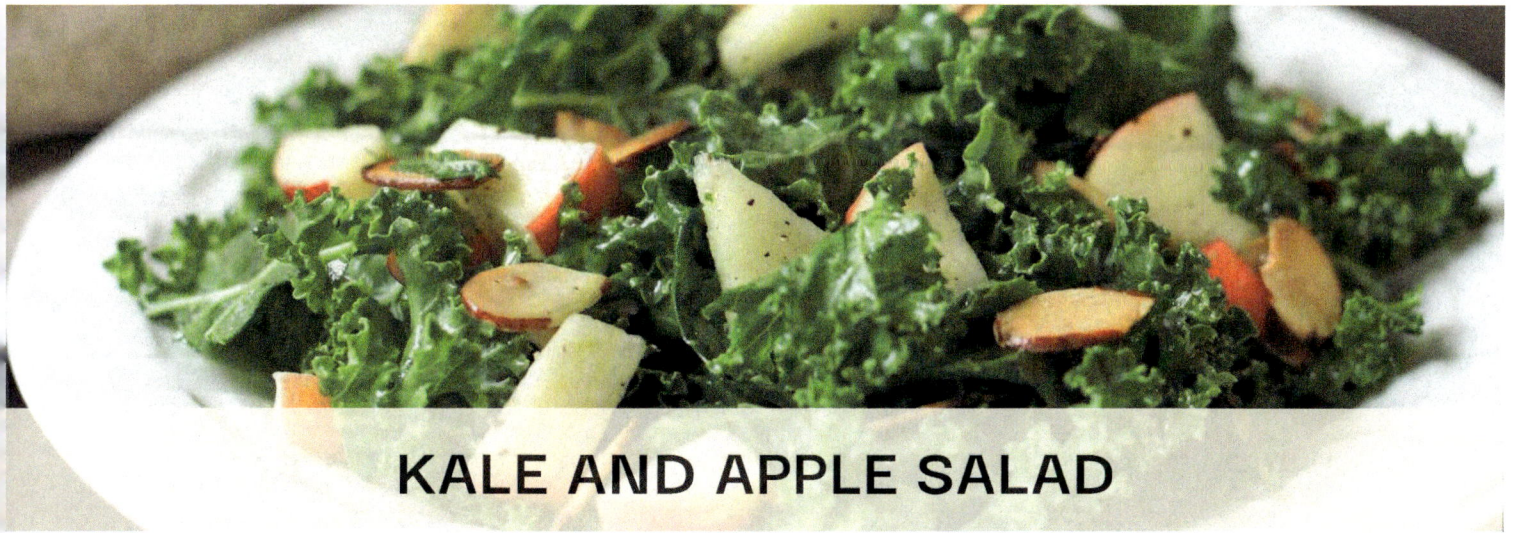

KALE AND APPLE SALAD

Kale and Apple Salad is a vibrant, crunchy, and refreshing dish that balances the earthy flavors of kale with the sweetness of apples. This salad is packed with nutrients and makes a perfect side dish or light meal, offering a delightful combination of textures and flavors.

Serves 	Preparation Time	Cooking Time
4	15 minutes	40 minute

Ingredients:

6 cups kale, chopped (stems removed)
1 large apple, thinly sliced
1/4 cup walnuts, toasted and chopped
1/4 cup dried cranberries
1/4 cup feta cheese, crumbled (optional)
2 tablespoons olive oil
1 tablespoon apple cider vinegar
1 teaspoon honey or maple syrup
Salt and black pepper to taste

Instructions:

1. **Prepare the Kale:** Place the chopped kale in a large bowl. Drizzle with a small amount of olive oil and a pinch of salt. Massage the kale with your hands for 2-3 minutes until it softens and turns a deeper green.
2. **Make the Dressing:** In a small bowl, whisk together the olive oil, apple cider vinegar, honey (or maple syrup), salt, and black pepper until well combined.
3. **Assemble the Salad:** Add the sliced apple, toasted walnuts, dried cranberries, and crumbled feta cheese (if using) to the massaged kale. Pour the dressing over the salad and toss everything together until evenly coated.
4. **Serve:** Serve the salad immediately or refrigerate it for 10-15 minutes to allow the flavors to meld together. Enjoy as a refreshing side dish or a light, healthy meal.

Nutrients (per serving)

Calories: 180 Sodium: 150 mg Carbohydrates: 16 g
Fiber: 4 g Protein: 4 g Calcium: 100 mg Fat: 12 g
Sugar: 9 g

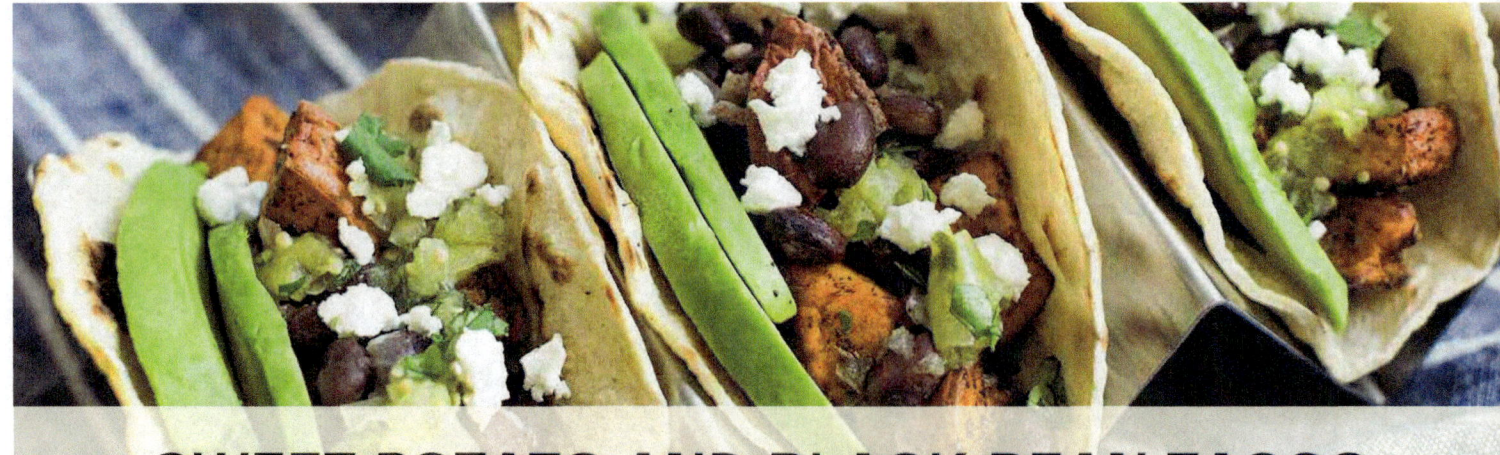

SWEET POTATO AND BLACK BEAN TACOS

Sweet Potato and Black Bean Tacos are a delicious and hearty option for a plant-based meal. The sweet, roasted potatoes pair perfectly with the savory black beans, all wrapped in a soft taco shell for a satisfying and flavorful dish.

Serves 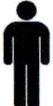	Preparation Time	Cooking Time 
4	10 minutes	30 minute

Ingredients:

- 2 medium sweet potatoes, peeled and diced
- 1 tablespoon olive oil
- 1 teaspoon ground cumin
- 1/2 teaspoon smoked paprika
- Salt and black pepper to taste
- 1 can (15 oz) black beans, drained and rinsed
- 1/2 cup red onion, finely chopped
- 1/4 cup fresh cilantro, chopped
- 8 small corn or whole wheat tortillas
- 1 avocado, sliced
- 1/4 cup crumbled feta cheese (optional)
- Lime wedges, for serving

Instructions:

1. **Roast the Sweet Potatoes:** Preheat your oven to 400°F (200°C). Toss the diced sweet potatoes with olive oil, ground cumin, smoked paprika, salt, and black pepper. Spread them out in a single layer on a baking sheet and roast for 25-30 minutes, or until tender and slightly caramelized, stirring halfway through.
2. **Prepare the Black Beans:** While the sweet potatoes are roasting, heat a skillet over medium heat. Add the black beans and cook until warmed through, about 5 minutes. Stir in the chopped red onion and cilantro, and season with a pinch of salt and pepper. Remove from heat.
3. **Assemble the Tacos:** Warm the tortillas in a dry skillet or microwave. To assemble, place a generous spoonful of roasted sweet potatoes onto each tortilla. Top with the black bean mixture, avocado slices, and crumbled feta cheese (if using).
4. **Serve:** Serve the tacos with lime wedges on the side for a fresh, tangy finish. Enjoy these flavorful tacos as a healthy, plant-based meal.

Nutrients (per serving)

Calories: 310 Sodium: 400 mg Carbohydrates: 50 g
Fiber: 12 g Protein: 9 g Calcium: 120 mg Fat: 9 g
Sugar: 7 g

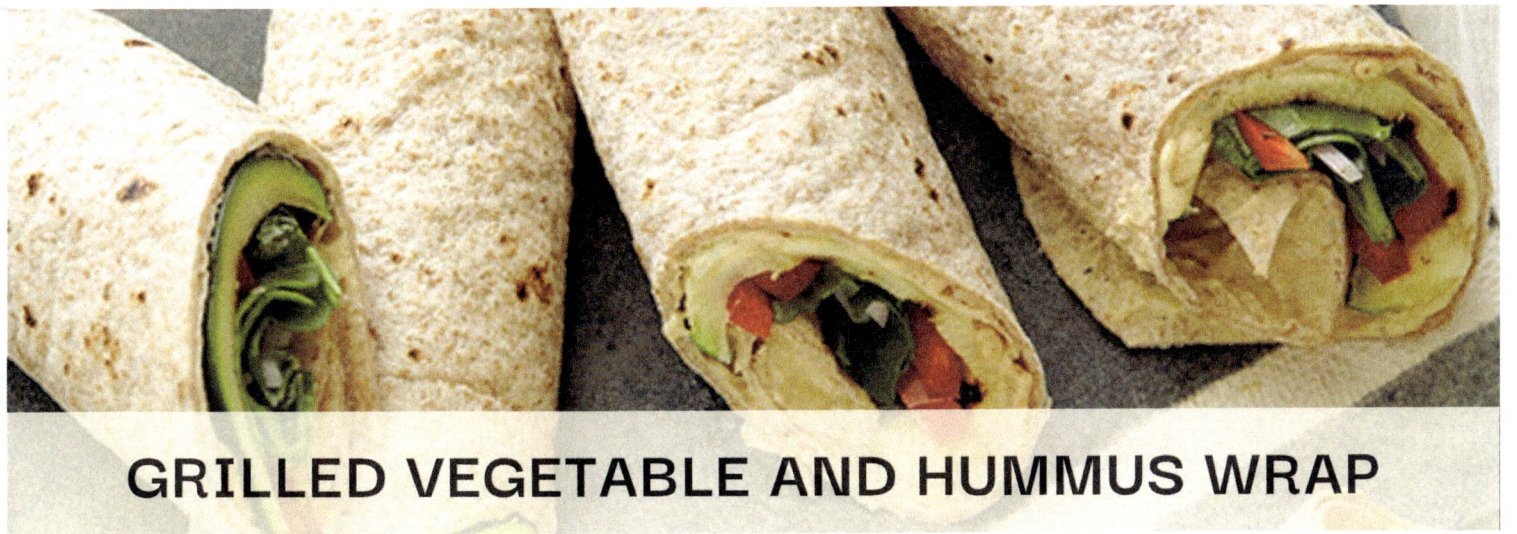

GRILLED VEGETABLE AND HUMMUS WRAP

Grilled Vegetable and Hummus Wrap is a healthy and flavorful option for a quick lunch or light dinner. Packed with a variety of grilled vegetables and creamy hummus, this wrap is both satisfying and nutrient-rich.

Serves	Preparation Time	Cooking Time
4	10 minutes	10 minute

Ingredients:

- 1 zucchini, sliced lengthwise
- 1 red bell pepper, sliced
- 1 yellow bell pepper, sliced
- 1 red onion, sliced into rings
- 1 tablespoon olive oil
- Salt and black pepper to taste
- 4 whole wheat tortillas or wraps
- 1/2 cup hummus (store-bought or homemade)
- 1/4 cup fresh spinach leaves
- 1/4 cup crumbled feta cheese (optional)

Instructions:

1. **Grill the Vegetables:** Preheat a grill or grill pan over medium-high heat. Toss the zucchini, bell peppers, and red onion slices with olive oil, salt, and black pepper. Grill the vegetables for 3-4 minutes on each side, or until they are tender and have nice grill marks. Remove from the grill and set aside.
2. **Assemble the Wraps:** Spread a generous amount of hummus over each tortilla. Layer with grilled vegetables, fresh spinach leaves, and crumbled feta cheese (if using).
3. **Wrap and Serve:** Roll up each tortilla tightly to form a wrap. Cut in half if desired, and serve immediately. Enjoy this wrap warm or at room temperature for a delicious and healthy meal.

Nutrients (per serving)

Calories: 270 Sodium: 450 mg Carbohydrates: 35 g

Fiber: 8 g Protein: 8 g Calcium: 100 mg Fat: 12 g

Sugar: 7 g

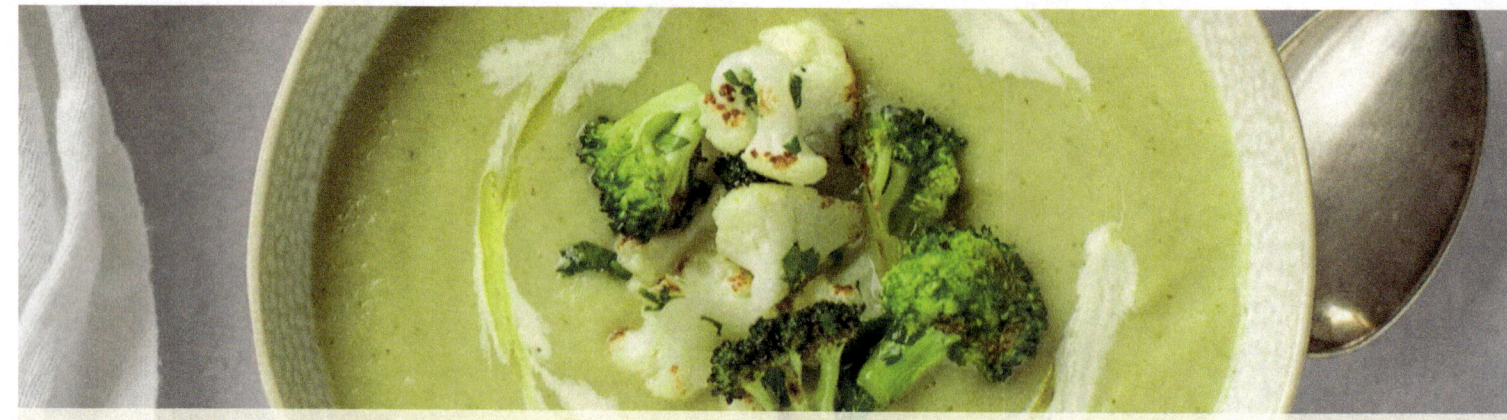

BROCCOLI AND CAULIFLOWER SOUP

Broccoli and Cauliflower Soup is a comforting and nutritious dish, perfect for a light meal or a warming appetizer. This creamy, vegetable-packed soup is both hearty and healthy, making it a great choice for those looking to enjoy a flavorful, wholesome bowl of goodness.

Serves 	Preparation Time	Cooking Time 
4	10 minutes	25 minute

Ingredients:

1 tablespoon olive oil
1 medium onion, chopped
2 cloves garlic, minced
4 cups broccoli florets
4 cups cauliflower florets
4 cups low-sodium vegetable broth
1 cup unsweetened almond milk (or any plant-based milk)
Salt and black pepper to taste
1/4 teaspoon ground nutmeg (optional)
1/4 cup nutritional yeast (optional, for a cheesy flavor)
Fresh parsley or chives, chopped, for garnish

Instructions:

1. **Sauté the Aromatics:** Heat olive oil in a large pot over medium heat. Add the chopped onion and sauté for 3-4 minutes, or until softened. Add the minced garlic and cook for an additional 1 minute until fragrant.
2. **Cook the Vegetables:** Add the broccoli and cauliflower florets to the pot. Pour in the vegetable broth, bringing the mixture to a boil. Reduce the heat to low, cover, and simmer for 15-20 minutes, or until the vegetables are tender.
3. **Blend the Soup:** Use an immersion blender to blend the soup until smooth and creamy. Alternatively, transfer the soup in batches to a blender and blend until smooth. Return the soup to the pot.
4. **Add Creaminess:** Stir in the almond milk, salt, black pepper, and ground nutmeg (if using). If desired, add nutritional yeast for a cheesy flavor. Heat the soup over low heat for an additional 5 minutes until warmed through.
5. **Serve:** Ladle the soup into bowls and garnish with fresh parsley or chives. Serve hot, accompanied by crusty bread or a light salad.

Nutrients (per serving)

Calories: 150 Sodium: 300 mg Carbohydrates: 18 g
Fiber: 6 g Protein: 6 g Calcium: 120 mg Fat: 6 g
Sugar: 4 g

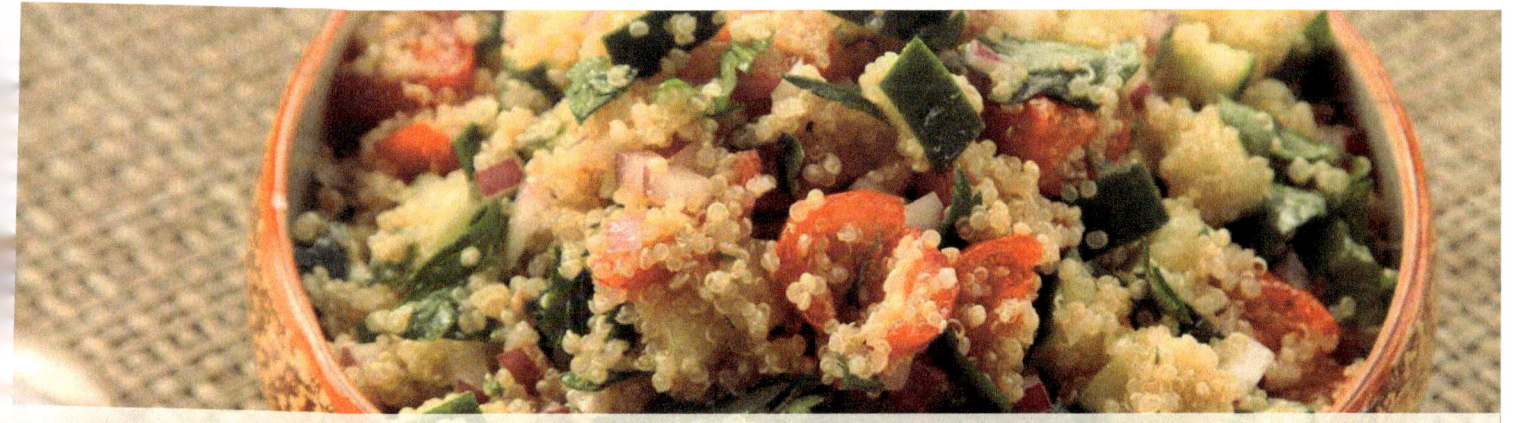

TOMATO AND CUCUMBER QUINOA SALAD

Tomato and Cucumber Quinoa Salad is a refreshing and nutritious dish that's perfect for a light lunch or as a side for dinner. The combination of juicy tomatoes, crisp cucumbers, and protein-rich quinoa creates a vibrant and satisfying salad that's both healthy and delicious.

Serves 	Preparation Time	Cooking Time 
4	10 minutes	15 minute

Ingredients:

1 cup quinoa, rinsed
2 cups water
1 cup cherry tomatoes, halved
1 cucumber, diced
1/4 cup red onion, finely chopped
1/4 cup fresh parsley, chopped
1/4 cup fresh basil, chopped (optional)
1/4 cup feta cheese, crumbled (optional)
2 tablespoons olive oil
1 tablespoon lemon juice
Salt and black pepper to taste

Instructions:

1. **Cook the Quinoa:** In a medium saucepan, combine the rinsed quinoa and water. Bring to a boil, then reduce the heat to low, cover, and simmer for 15 minutes, or until the quinoa is cooked and the water is absorbed. Fluff the quinoa with a fork and let it cool to room temperature.
2. **Prepare the Salad Ingredients:** In a large bowl, combine the cherry tomatoes, diced cucumber, red onion, and chopped parsley. If using, add the fresh basil and crumbled feta cheese.
3. **Assemble the Salad:** Add the cooled quinoa to the bowl with the vegetables. Drizzle with olive oil and lemon juice. Toss gently to combine, making sure all ingredients are evenly coated.
4. **Season and Serve:** Season with salt and black pepper to taste. Serve immediately or refrigerate for 30 minutes to let the flavors meld.

Nutrients (per serving)

Calories: 220 Sodium: 180 mg Carbohydrates: 28 g
Fiber: 4 g Protein: 6 g Calcium: 80 mg Fat: 9 g
Sugar: 4 g

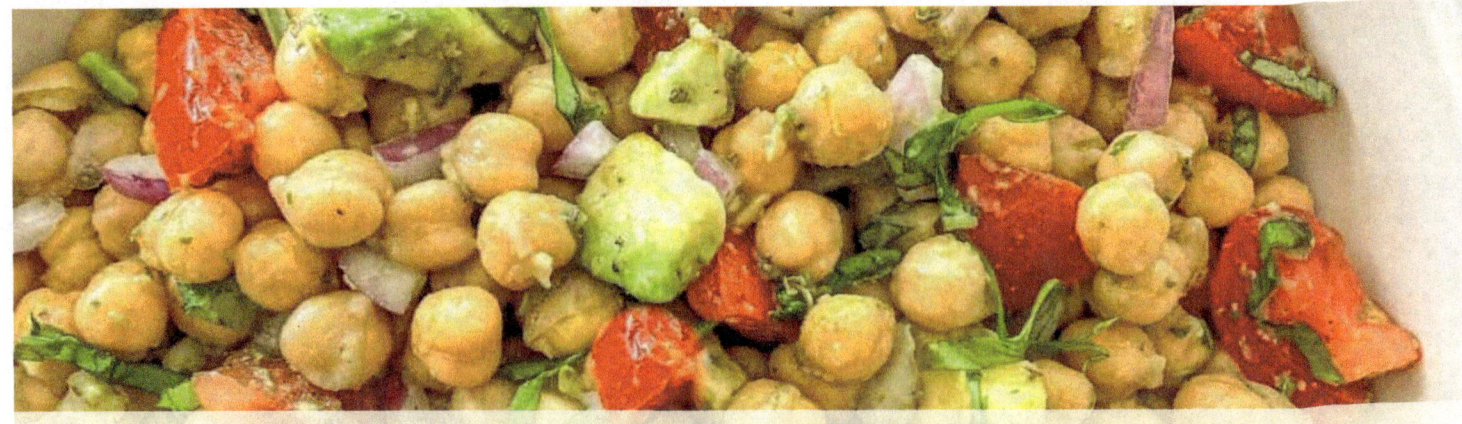

CHICKPEA AND AVOCADO SALAD

Chickpea and Avocado Salad is a creamy, protein-packed dish that's full of vibrant flavors and healthy ingredients. This salad is perfect for a quick lunch or as a refreshing side dish, offering a great balance of textures and nutrients.

Serves	Preparation Time	Cooking Time
4	10 minutes	0 minute

Ingredients:

- 1 can (15 oz) chickpeas, drained and rinsed
- 1 large avocado, diced
- 1 cup cherry tomatoes, halved
- 1/2 cucumber, diced
- 1/4 red onion, finely chopped
- 2 tablespoons fresh cilantro, chopped
- 2 tablespoons olive oil
- 1 tablespoon lime juice
- Salt and black pepper to taste

Instructions:

1. **Prepare the Ingredients:b** In a large bowl, combine the drained chickpeas, diced avocado, cherry tomatoes, cucumber, and red onion.
2. **Mix the Salad:** Add the chopped cilantro, olive oil, and lime juice to the bowl. Gently toss all the ingredients together until well combined.
3. **Season and Serve:** Season the salad with salt and black pepper to taste. Serve immediately or chill in the refrigerator for about 15 minutes to let the flavors meld.

Nutrients (per serving)

Calories: 230 Sodium: 210 mg Carbohydrates: 20 g
Fiber: 8 g Protein: 6 g Calcium: 40 mg Fat: 15 g
Sugar: 3 g

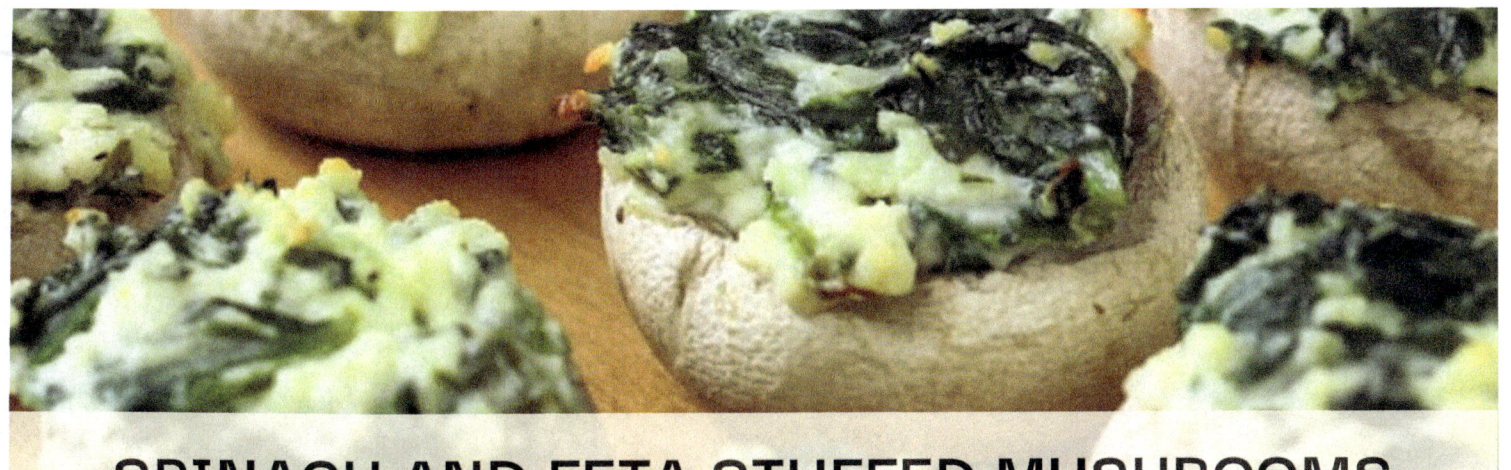

SPINACH AND FETA STUFFED MUSHROOMS

Spinach and Feta Stuffed Mushrooms are a savory, bite-sized treat perfect for appetizers or as a side dish. The combination of earthy mushrooms, creamy feta, and nutritious spinach makes this dish both flavorful and healthy.

Serves 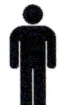	Preparation Time	Cooking Time 
4	15 minutes	20 minute

Ingredients:

12 large white mushrooms, stems removed and finely chopped
1 tablespoon olive oil
1/2 onion, finely chopped
2 garlic cloves, minced
2 cups fresh spinach, chopped
1/2 cup feta cheese, crumbled
1/4 cup breadcrumbs (optional for added texture)
1/4 teaspoon black pepper
1/4 teaspoon salt

Instructions:

1. **Preheat the Oven:** Preheat your oven to 375°F (190°C).
2. **Prepare the Mushroom Caps:** Clean the mushroom caps with a damp cloth and set them aside.
3. **Cook the Filling:** Heat olive oil in a skillet over medium heat. Add the chopped onion and garlic, sautéing until softened, about 2-3 minutes. Add the chopped mushroom stems and spinach to the skillet. Cook until the spinach wilts and the liquid from the mushrooms evaporates, about 4-5 minutes. Remove the skillet from the heat and stir in the feta cheese, breadcrumbs (if using), black pepper, and salt.
4. **Stuff the Mushrooms:** Spoon the spinach and feta mixture into each mushroom cap, pressing down slightly to ensure they're well-filled.
5. **Bake:** Arrange the stuffed mushrooms on a baking sheet. Bake in the preheated oven for 15-20 minutes, or until the mushrooms are tender and the tops are lightly golden.
6. **Serve:** Allow the stuffed mushrooms to cool slightly before serving. Enjoy them warm as a delicious appetizer or side dish.

Nutrients (per serving)

Calories: 150 Sodium: 300 mg Carbohydrates: 8 g
Fiber: 2 g Protein: 6 g Calcium: 130 mg Fat: 10 g
Sugar: 2 g

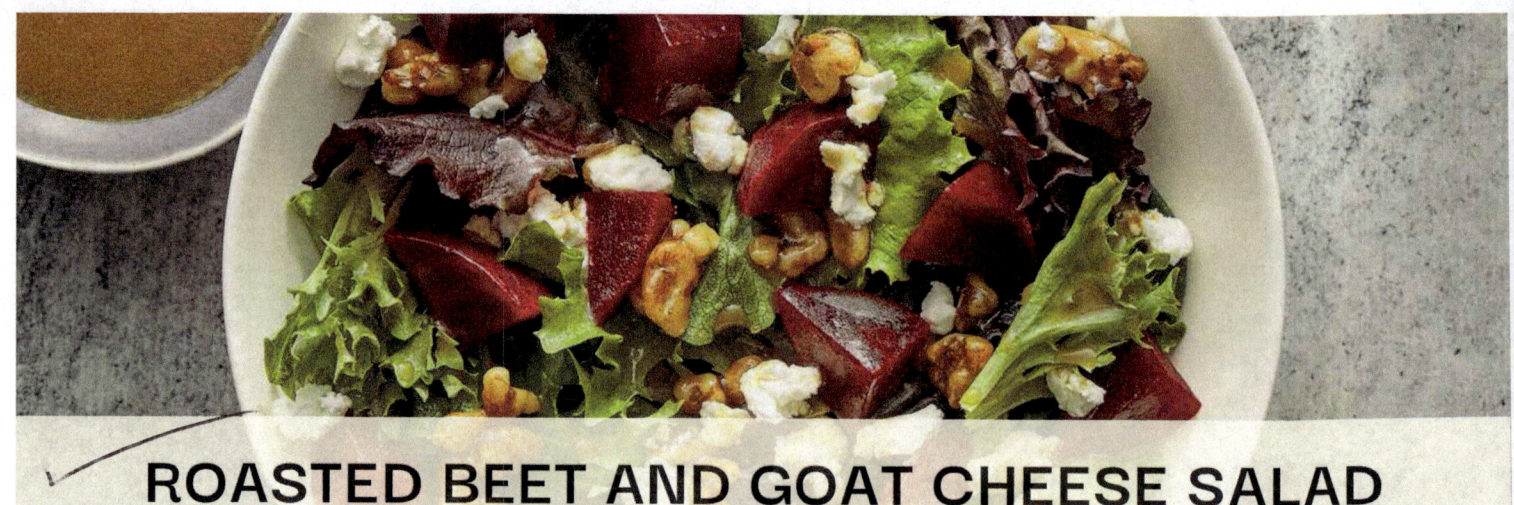

ROASTED BEET AND GOAT CHEESE SALAD

Roasted Beet and Goat Cheese Salad is a vibrant and nutritious dish, combining the earthy sweetness of roasted beets with the creamy tang of goat cheese. It's a perfect blend of flavors and textures, ideal for a light lunch or as a starter.

Serves	Preparation Time	Cooking Time
4	10 minutes	55 minute

Ingredients:

4 medium beets, trimmed and scrubbed
2 tablespoons olive oil, divided
4 cups mixed greens (like arugula, spinach, or spring mix)
1/2 cup goat cheese, crumbled
1/4 cup walnuts, toasted and chopped
2 tablespoons balsamic vinegar
1 teaspoon honey (optional)
Salt and black pepper to taste

Instructions:

1. **Roast the Beets:** Preheat your oven to 400°F (200°C). Wrap each beet individually in aluminum foil and place them on a baking sheet. Roast for 45-60 minutes, or until the beets are tender when pierced with a fork. Once roasted, remove the beets from the oven, let them cool slightly, then peel and slice them into wedges.
2. **Prepare the Dressing:** In a small bowl, whisk together 1 tablespoon of olive oil, balsamic vinegar, honey (if using), salt, and black pepper.
3. **Assemble the Salad:** In a large bowl, toss the mixed greens with the remaining tablespoon of olive oil.
4. Arrange the roasted beet wedges on top of the greens. Sprinkle the crumbled goat cheese and toasted walnuts over the salad.
5. **Serve:** Drizzle the salad with the prepared dressing. Serve immediately and enjoy this fresh, flavorful salad.

Nutrients (per serving)

Calories: 210 Sodium: 220 mg Carbohydrates: 14 g
Fiber: 4 g Protein: 7 g Calcium: 80 mg Fat: 15 g
Sugar: 9 g

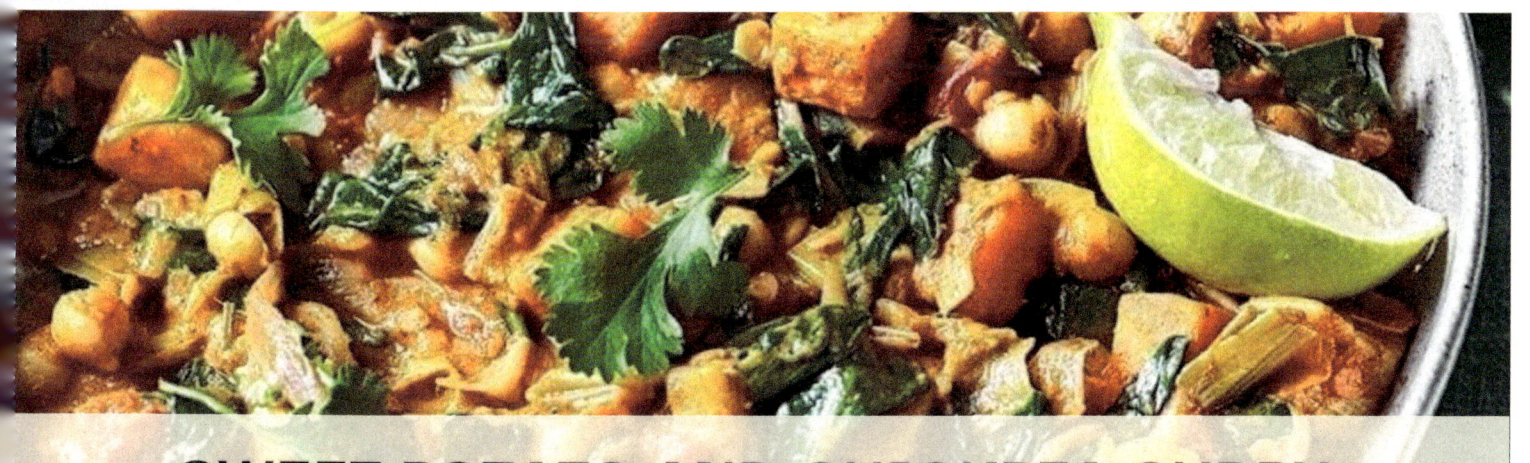

SWEET POTATO AND CHICKPEA CURRY

Sweet Potato and Chickpea Curry is a hearty, flavorful dish that combines the natural sweetness of sweet potatoes with the satisfying texture of chickpeas. It's a comforting meal that's rich in nutrients and perfect for a wholesome dinner.

Serves 	Preparation Time	Cooking Time 
4	15 minutes	30 minute

Ingredients:

2 tablespoons olive oil
1 onion, finely chopped
3 garlic cloves, minced
1 tablespoon ginger, minced
2 tablespoons curry powder
1 teaspoon ground cumin
1 teaspoon ground turmeric
1/2 teaspoon ground cinnamon
2 medium sweet potatoes, peeled and cubed
1 can (15 oz) chickpeas, drained and rinsed
1 can (14 oz) diced tomatoes
1 can (14 oz) coconut milk
1 cup vegetable broth
Salt and black pepper to taste
Fresh cilantro, chopped (for garnish)

Instructions:

1. **Cook the Aromatics:** Heat the olive oil in a large pot over medium heat. Add the chopped onion and sauté until soft and translucent, about 5 minutes.
2. Stir in the garlic and ginger, cooking until fragrant, about 1-2 minutes.
3. **Add the Spices:** Add the curry powder, ground cumin, ground turmeric, and ground cinnamon to the pot. Stir well to coat the onions, garlic, and ginger with the spices, and cook for another 1-2 minutes to enhance the flavors.
4. **Simmer the Curry:** Add the cubed sweet potatoes, chickpeas, diced tomatoes, coconut milk, and vegetable broth to the pot. Stir well to combine all ingredients. Bring the mixture to a boil, then reduce the heat to low. Cover the pot and simmer for 20-25 minutes, or until the sweet potatoes are tender and the flavors have melded together.
5. **Season and Serve:** Season the curry with salt and black pepper to taste. Serve hot, garnished with fresh cilantro.

Nutrients (per serving)

Calories: 320 Sodium: 380 mg Carbohydrates: 45 g
Fiber: 8 g Protein: 8 g Calcium: 80 mg Fat: 14 g
Sugar: 9 g

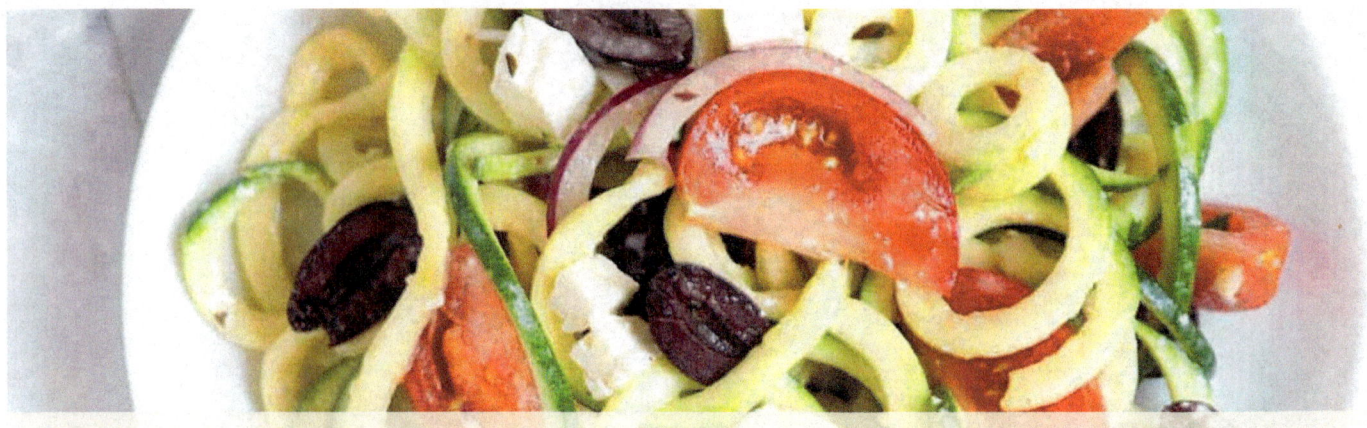

MEDITERRANEAN ZOODLE SALAD

Mediterranean Zoodle Salad is a light and refreshing dish that combines the vibrant flavors of the Mediterranean with the healthy twist of zucchini noodles. This salad is perfect for a quick, nutritious meal that's low in carbs and full of fresh, colorful vegetables.

Serves 	**Preparation Time**	**Cooking Time** 
4	15 minutes	0 minute

Ingredients:

4 medium zucchini, spiralized into noodles (zoodles)
1 cup cherry tomatoes, halved
1/2 cup Kalamata olives, pitted and sliced
1/2 red onion, thinly sliced
1/2 cup cucumber, diced
1/2 cup feta cheese, crumbled
1/4 cup fresh parsley, chopped
2 tablespoons extra-virgin olive oil
1 tablespoon lemon juice
1 teaspoon dried oregano
Salt and black pepper to taste

Instructions:

1. **Prepare the Zoodles:** Spiralize the zucchini into noodles using a spiralizer. If you don't have a spiralizer, you can use a julienne peeler or a regular vegetable peeler to create thin strips.
2. **Mix the Vegetables:** In a large bowl, combine the zoodles, cherry tomatoes, Kalamata olives, red onion, and cucumber. Toss gently to mix the ingredients evenly.
3. **Make the Dressing:** In a small bowl, whisk together the extra-virgin olive oil, lemon juice, dried oregano, salt, and black pepper.
4. **Assemble the Salad:** Pour the dressing over the zoodle mixture and toss until the zoodles and vegetables are well coated.
5. **Serve:** Transfer the salad to a serving platter. Sprinkle the crumbled feta cheese and chopped parsley over the top. Serve immediately.

Nutrients (per serving)

Calories: 160 Sodium: 360 mg Carbohydrates: 9 g
Fiber: 3 g Protein: 5 g Calcium: 120 mg Fat: 12 g
Sugar: 5 g

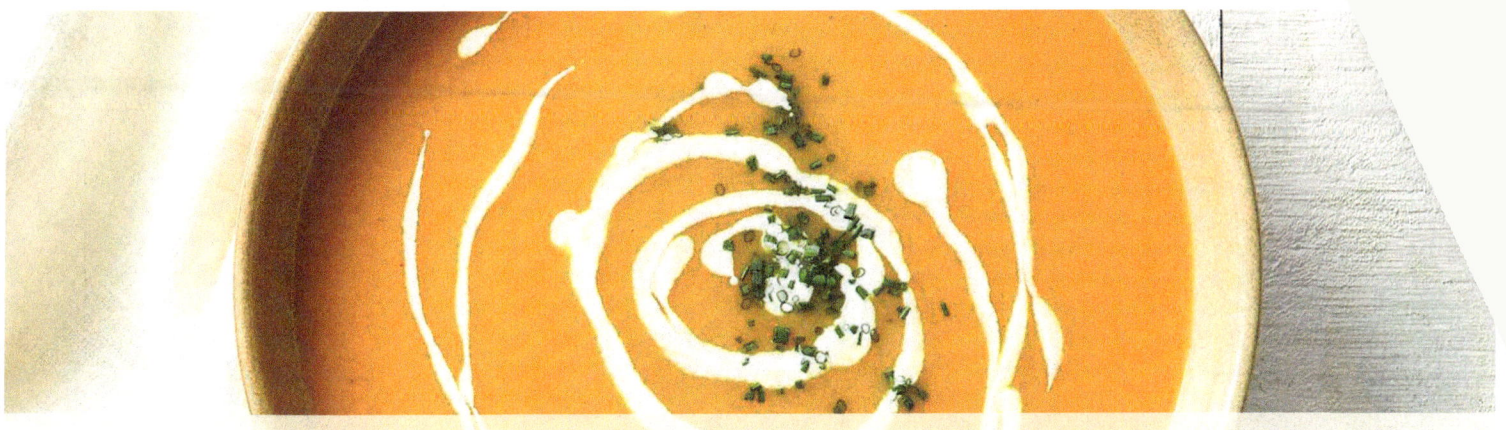

ROASTED BUTTERNUT SQUASH SOUP

Roasted Butternut Squash Soup is a creamy and comforting dish that's perfect for chilly days. This flavorful soup highlights the natural sweetness of butternut squash, enhanced by roasting, and is blended to create a smooth, velvety texture.

Serves 	Preparation Time	Cooking Time 
4	15 minutes	45 minute

Ingredients:

1 large butternut squash, peeled, seeded, and cubed
2 tablespoons olive oil
Salt and black pepper to taste
1 onion, chopped
3 garlic cloves, minced
4 cups vegetable broth
1/2 teaspoon ground nutmeg
1/2 teaspoon ground cinnamon
1/2 cup coconut milk or heavy cream (optional)
Fresh thyme or parsley for garnish (optional)

Instructions:

1. **Roast the Butternut Squash:** Preheat the oven to 400°F (200°C). Place the cubed butternut squash on a baking sheet. Drizzle with 1 tablespoon of olive oil, and season with salt and black pepper. Toss to coat evenly. Roast in the oven for 25-30 minutes, or until the squash is tender and lightly browned.
2. **Cook the Aromatics:** In a large pot, heat the remaining 1 tablespoon of olive oil over medium heat. Add the chopped onion and sauté until soft and translucent, about 5 minutes. Add the minced garlic and cook for another 1-2 minutes until fragrant.
3. **Simmer the Soup:** Add the roasted butternut squash to the pot along with the vegetable broth, ground nutmeg, and ground cinnamon. Stir well to combine. Bring the mixture to a boil, then reduce the heat to low. Cover and simmer for 15-20 minutes to allow the flavors to meld.
4. **Blend the Soup:** Use an immersion blender to blend the soup until smooth and creamy. If you don't have an immersion blender, carefully transfer the soup in batches to a countertop blender. If using, stir in the coconut milk or heavy cream to add extra creaminess.
5. **Serve:** Taste and adjust seasoning with more salt and pepper if needed. Ladle the soup into bowls, garnish with fresh thyme or parsley if desired, and serve hot.

Nutrients (per serving)

Calories: 180 Sodium: 450 mg Carbohydrates: 24 g
Fiber: 6 g Protein: 3 g Calcium: 90 mg Fat: 8 g
Sugar: 7 g

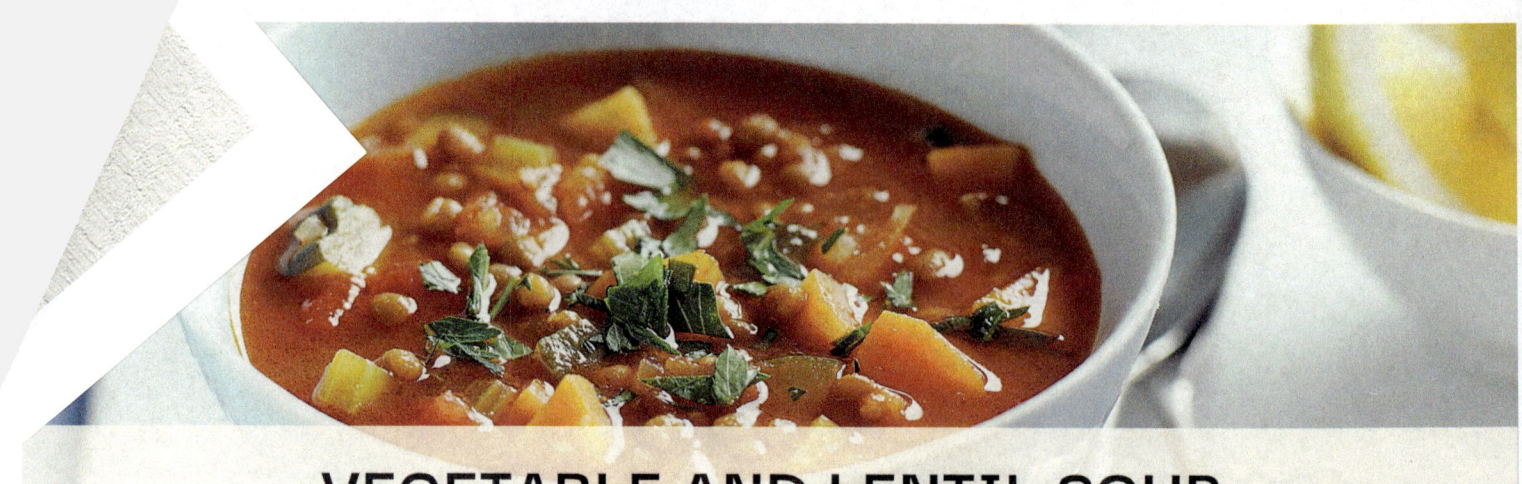

VEGETABLE AND LENTIL SOUP

Vegetable and Lentil Soup is a hearty and nutritious dish, perfect for a wholesome meal. Packed with protein-rich lentils and a variety of vegetables, this soup is not only filling but also rich in flavor and nutrients.

Serves		Preparation Time		Cooking Time	
~~4~~ 5. 176c		15 minutes		45 minute	

Ingredients:

- 1 cup green or brown lentils, rinsed
- 1 onion, chopped
- ~~2~~ 3 carrots, sliced
- 2 celery stalks, chopped
- 2 garlic cloves, minced
- ~~1 zucchini, diced~~
- 1 cup spinach or kale, chopped
- 1 can (14.5 oz) diced tomatoes, with juice
- 6 cups vegetable broth
- 1 tablespoon olive oil
- 1 teaspoon dried thyme
- 1 teaspoon ground cumin
- 1 bay leaf
- Salt and black pepper to taste
- Fresh parsley for garnish (optional)

Instructions:

1. **Prepare the Base:** Heat olive oil in a large pot over medium heat. Add the chopped onion, carrots, and celery. Sauté until the vegetables are softened, about 5-7 minutes. Add the minced garlic and cook for another 1-2 minutes until fragrant.
2. **Add Lentils and Spices:** Stir in the rinsed lentils, dried thyme, ground cumin, and bay leaf. Mix well to coat the lentils with the spices.
3. **Simmer the Soup:** Add the vegetable broth and diced tomatoes (with juice) to the pot. Stir to combine. Bring the mixture to a boil, then reduce the heat to low. Cover and simmer for 25-30 minutes, or until the lentils are tender.
4. **Add the Vegetables:** Stir in the diced zucchini and chopped spinach or kale. Continue to cook for another 10 minutes, until the vegetables are tender.
5. **Season and Serve:** Remove the bay leaf. Taste the soup and adjust the seasoning with salt and black pepper as needed. Ladle the soup into bowls, garnish with fresh parsley if desired, and serve hot.

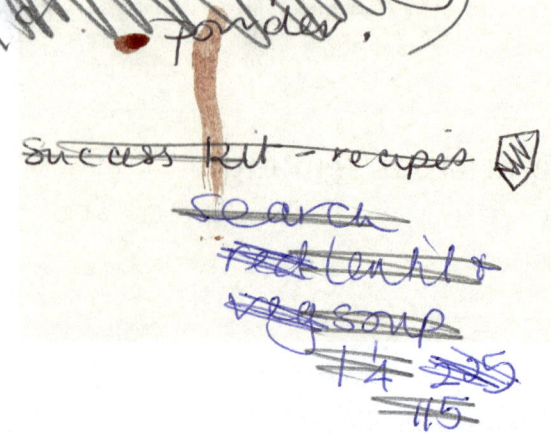

Nutrients (per serving)

Calories: 220 Sodium: 500 mg Carbohydrates: 35 g

Fiber: 12 g Protein: 12 g Calcium: 80 mg Fat: 4 g

Sugar: 7 g

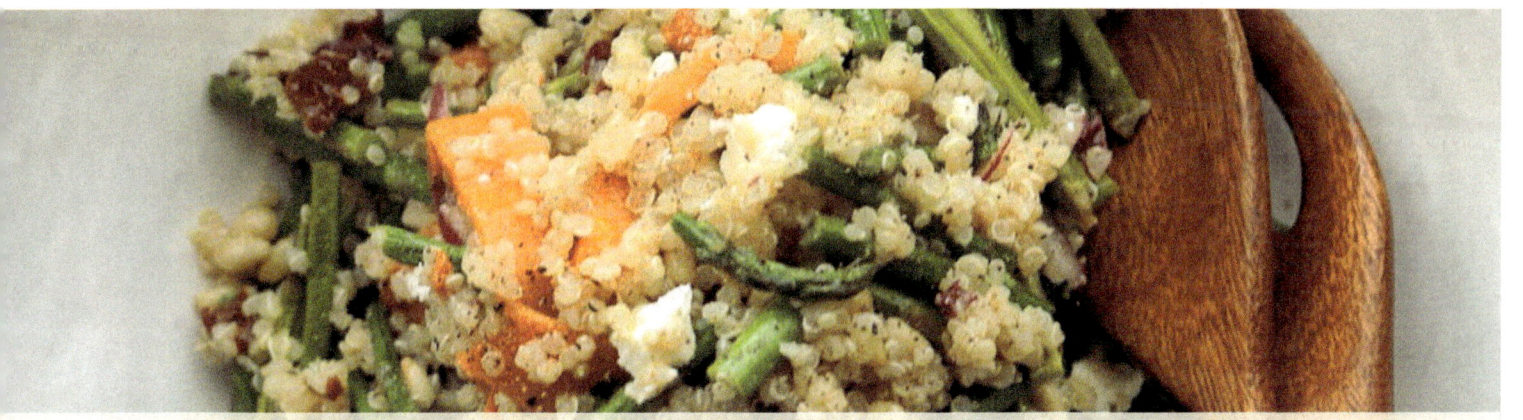

GRILLED ASPARAGUS AND QUINOA SALAD

Grilled Asparagus and Quinoa Salad is a light yet satisfying dish that combines the nutty flavor of quinoa with the smokiness of grilled asparagus. It's a perfect meal for a healthy lunch or dinner.

Serves	Preparation Time	Cooking Time 
4	10 minutes	20 minute

Ingredients:

1 cup quinoa, rinsed
1 bunch asparagus, trimmed
2 tablespoons olive oil, divided
1 lemon, juiced
1 garlic clove, minced
1/4 cup feta cheese, crumbled
1/4 cup cherry tomatoes, halved
2 tablespoons fresh parsley, chopped
Salt and black pepper to taste

Instructions:

1. **Cook the Quinoa:** In a medium saucepan, combine quinoa with 2 cups of water. Bring to a boil, then reduce the heat to low, cover, and simmer for 15 minutes or until the water is absorbed. Fluff with a fork and set aside to cool.
2. **Grill the Asparagus:** Preheat a grill or grill pan over medium-high heat.
3. Toss the asparagus with 1 tablespoon of olive oil, and season with salt and pepper. Grill the asparagus for 5-7 minutes, turning occasionally until tender and slightly charred. Remove from the grill and cut into 2-inch pieces.
4. **Prepare the Dressing:** In a small bowl, whisk together the remaining 1 tablespoon of olive oil, lemon juice, and minced garlic. Season with salt and pepper to taste.
5. **Assemble the Salad:** In a large bowl, combine the cooked quinoa, grilled asparagus, cherry tomatoes, and fresh parsley. Drizzle with the lemon-garlic dressing and toss to combine. Gently fold in the crumbled feta cheese.
6. **Serve:** Transfer the salad to a serving platter or individual bowls. Serve immediately, or chill in the refrigerator for 30 minutes for a cold salad.

Nutrients (per serving)

Calories: 240 Sodium: 220 mg Carbohydrates: 28 g
Fiber: 5 g Protein: 8 g Calcium: 80 mg Fat: 10 g
Sugar: 3 g

AFTERNOON MEAL

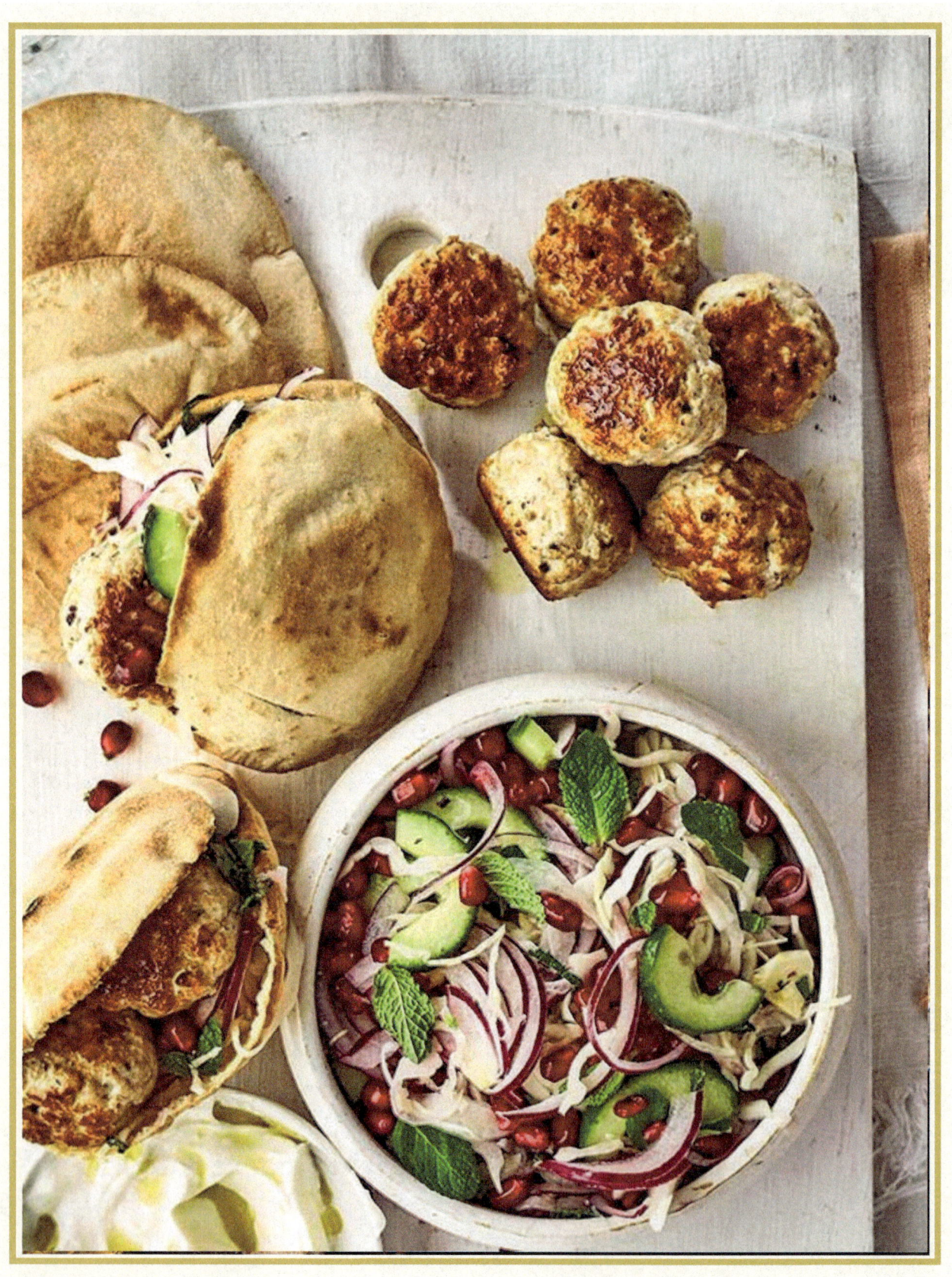

TABLE OF CONTENTS

- Grilled Tofu with Stir-Fried Vegetables (Green) — 54
- Vegetable and Hummus Wrap (Green) — 55
- Chickpea and Spinach Stir-Fry (Green) — 56
- Roasted Sweet Potatoes with Cinnamon (Green) — 57
- Cauliflower and Lentil Stew (Green) — 58
- Broccoli and Kale Salad (Green) — 59
- Mixed Greens with Citrus Vinaigrette (Green) — 60
- Sautéed Zucchini with Tomatoes (Green) — 61
- Balsamic Roasted Vegetables (Green) — 62
- Quinoa and Roasted Vegetable Bowl (Green) — 63
- Zucchini Noodles with Marinara Sauce (Green) — 64
- Stuffed Zucchini Boats (Green) — 65
- Cabbage and Apple Slaw (Green) — 66
- Grilled Portobello Mushrooms (Green) — 67
- Spinach and Quinoa Stuffed Peppers (Green) — 68
- Butternut Squash and Sage Risotto (Green) — 69
- Roasted Cauliflower Tacos (Green) — 70
- Zoodle and Pesto Salad (Green) — 71
- Eggplant and Tomato Gratin (Green)
- Grilled Peppers and Onions (Green)

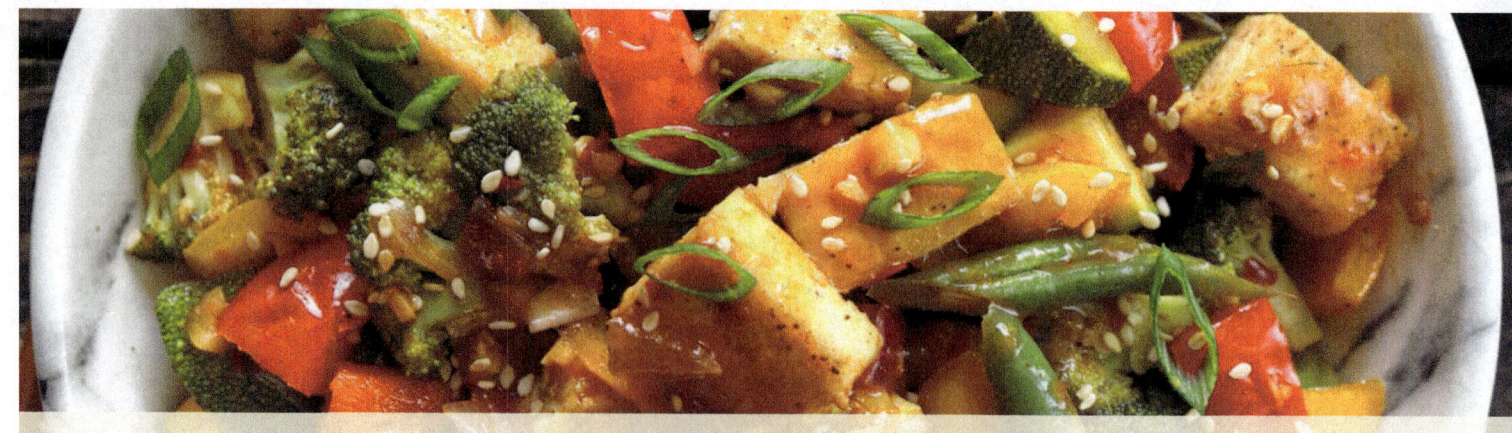

GRILLED TOFU WITH STIR-FRIED VEGETABLES

Grilled Tofu with Stir-Fried Vegetables is a balanced and protein-rich dish that pairs the smoky flavor of grilled tofu with the freshness of stir-fried vegetables. It's a satisfying and nutritious meal, perfect for a plant-based diet.

Serves	Preparation Time	Cooking Time 
4	15 minutes	20 minute

Ingredients:

- 1 block firm tofu, pressed and cut into slices
- 2 tablespoons soy sauce (or tamari for gluten-free)
- 1 tablespoon olive oil
- 1 red bell pepper, sliced
- 1 zucchini, sliced
- 1 carrot, julienned
- 1 cup broccoli florets
- 2 garlic cloves, minced
- 1 tablespoon sesame oil
- 2 tablespoons low-sodium soy sauce
- 1 tablespoon rice vinegar
- 1 teaspoon sesame seeds
- Salt and black pepper to taste
- Fresh cilantro for garnish (optional)

Instructions:

1. **Marinate the Tofu:** In a small bowl, mix 2 tablespoons of soy sauce with 1 tablespoon of olive oil. Place the tofu slices in a shallow dish and pour the marinade over them, ensuring each slice is well coated. Let it marinate for at least 15 minutes.
2. **Grill the Tofu:** Preheat a grill or grill pan over medium heat. Grill the tofu slices for about 4-5 minutes on each side, until they are golden brown and have grill marks. Set aside.
3. **Stir-Fry the Vegetables:** Heat sesame oil in a large skillet or wok over medium-high heat. Add the minced garlic and stir-fry for 30 seconds until fragrant. Add the broccoli florets, carrot, and zucchini. Stir-fry for 3-4 minutes until the vegetables are tender-crisp. Add the sliced red bell pepper and stir-fry for another 2 minutes.
4. **Season the Vegetables:** Stir in the remaining soy sauce and rice vinegar. Toss the vegetables to coat them evenly in the sauce. Season with salt and black pepper to taste.
5. **Assemble the Dish:** Arrange the grilled tofu slices on a serving plate. Top with the stir-fried vegetables and sprinkle with sesame seeds. Garnish with fresh cilantro if desired.
6. **Serve:** Serve hot, either as a standalone dish or with a side of steamed rice or quinoa.

Nutrients (per serving)

Calories: 210 Sodium: 450 mg Carbohydrates: 10 g
Fiber: 3 g Protein: 12 g Calcium: 150 mg Fat: 14 g
Sugar: 4 g

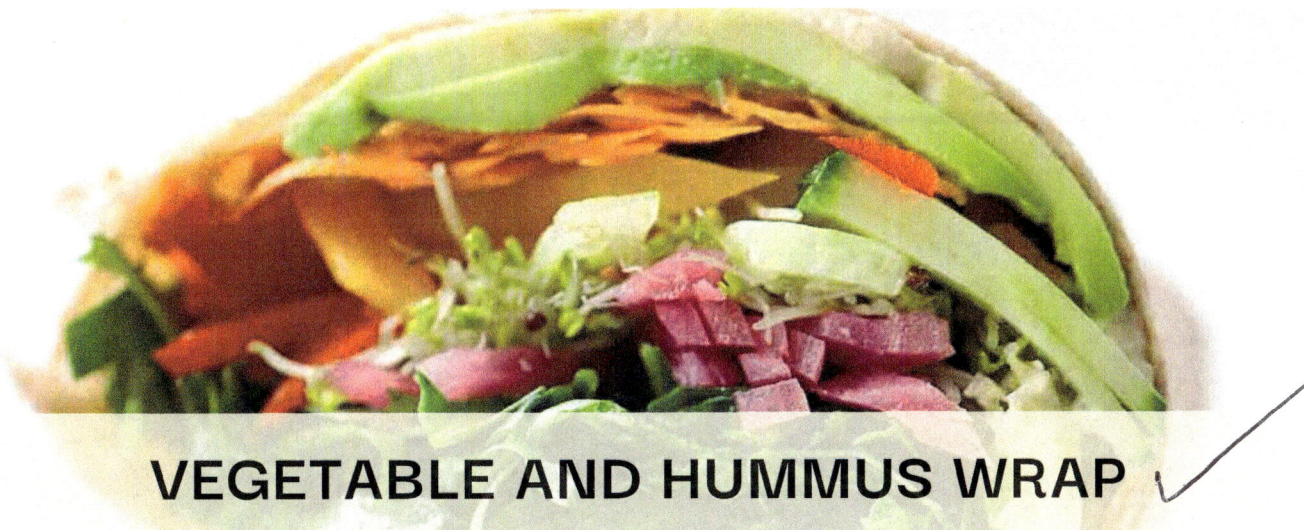

VEGETABLE AND HUMMUS WRAP ✓

The Vegetable and Hummus Wrap is a fresh, crunchy, and nutritious meal option, perfect for a quick lunch or light dinner. Packed with colorful veggies and creamy hummus, this wrap is both satisfying and healthy.

Serves	Preparation Time	Cooking Time
4	10 minutes	5 minute

Ingredients:

- 4 whole wheat or gluten-free tortillas 1
- 1 cup hummus (store-bought or homemade) ¼ *or cream cheese*
- 1 red bell pepper, thinly sliced ¼
- 1 cucumber, julienned *slice*
- 1 carrot, julienned ¼
- 1 avocado, sliced ¼ 1
- 1 cup baby spinach leaves ¼
- 1/4 cup red onion, thinly sliced *slice*
- 2 tablespoons feta cheese (optional) ½
- Salt and pepper to taste
- 1 tablespoon olive oil (optional for grilling)

avo or feta

Instructions:

1. **Prepare the Vegetables:** Wash and slice all vegetables (red bell pepper, cucumber, carrot, avocado, and red onion). Set aside the baby spinach leaves.
2. **Assemble the Wrap:** Lay each tortilla flat on a clean surface. Spread about 1/4 cup of hummus evenly over the center of each tortilla. Layer the spinach leaves, sliced bell pepper, cucumber, carrot, avocado, and red onion on top of the hummus. Sprinkle with feta cheese if using, and season with salt and pepper to taste.
3. **Roll the Wrap:** Fold in the sides of the tortilla, then tightly roll it up from the bottom to the top, ensuring all the fillings are enclosed.
4. **Optional Grilling:** If you prefer a warm wrap, lightly brush each wrap with olive oil and grill on a pan over medium heat for 2-3 minutes on each side until the tortilla is golden and crispy.
5. **Serve:** Slice each wrap in half and serve immediately. These wraps are perfect for dipping in extra hummus or enjoying with a side salad.

Nutrients (per serving)

Calories: 250 Sodium: 350 mg Carbohydrates: 30 g
Fiber: 8 g Protein: 7 g Calcium: 60 mg Fat: 12 g
Sugar: 4 g

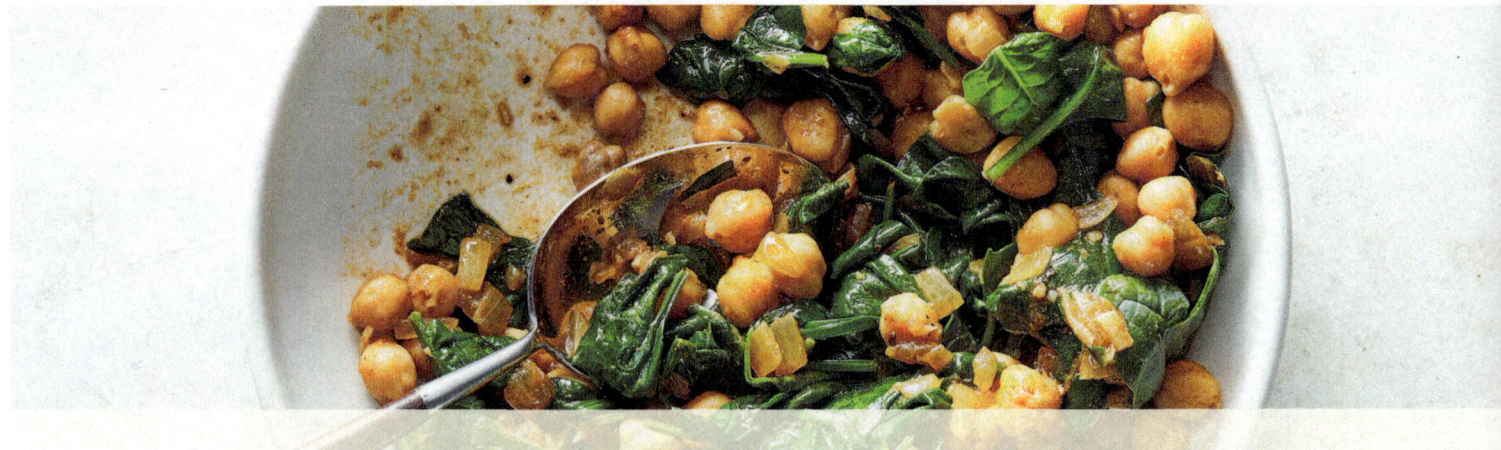

CHICKPEA AND SPINACH STIR-FRY

Chickpea and Spinach Stir-Fry is a quick and nutritious dish featuring protein-packed chickpeas and vibrant spinach. It's a flavorful, one-pan meal that's perfect for a healthy lunch or dinner.

Serves 	Preparation Time	Cooking Time 
4	10 minutes	15 minute

Ingredients:

1 can (15 oz) chickpeas, drained and rinsed
2 tablespoons olive oil
1 onion, diced
2 garlic cloves, minced
1 bell pepper, sliced
1 cup cherry tomatoes, halved
4 cups fresh spinach
1 teaspoon ground cumin
1/2 teaspoon paprika
1/4 teaspoon turmeric
Salt and black pepper to taste
1 tablespoon lemon juice
Fresh parsley for garnish (optional)

Instructions:

1. **Prepare the Ingredients:** Drain and rinse the chickpeas. Slice the bell pepper and halve the cherry tomatoes. Mince the garlic and dice the onion.
2. **Cook the Aromatics:** Heat olive oil in a large skillet over medium heat. Add the diced onion and cook for 3-4 minutes until it becomes translucent. Stir in the minced garlic and cook for an additional 30 seconds until fragrant.
3. **Add Vegetables and Spices:** Add the sliced bell pepper and cherry tomatoes to the skillet. Cook for 4-5 minutes until the vegetables start to soften. Stir in the ground cumin, paprika, turmeric, salt, and black pepper.
4. **Incorporate Chickpeas and Spinach:** Add the chickpeas to the skillet and cook for 2-3 minutes until heated through. Stir in the fresh spinach and cook until wilted, about 1-2 minutes.
5. **Finish and Serve:** Remove from heat and drizzle with lemon juice. Garnish with fresh parsley if desired. Serve hot as a main dish or alongside your favorite grain.

Nutrients (per serving)

Calories: 220 Sodium: 300 mg Carbohydrates: 30 g
Fiber: 8 g Protein: 10 g Calcium: 120 mg Fat: 8 g
Sugar: 6 g

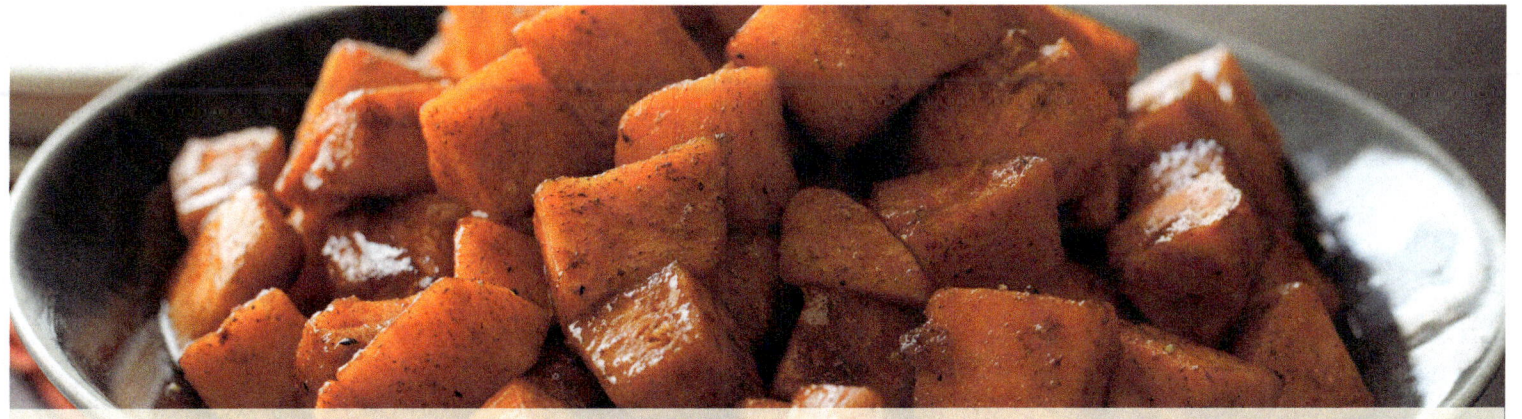

ROASTED SWEET POTATOES WITH CINNAMON

Roasted Sweet Potatoes with Cinnamon is a delightful side dish that combines the natural sweetness of sweet potatoes with aromatic cinnamon. This dish is simple to prepare and makes for a comforting and nutritious addition to any meal.

Serves	Preparation Time	Cooking Time
4	10 minutes	30 minute

Ingredients:

4 medium sweet potatoes, peeled and cut into cubes
2 tablespoons olive oil
1 teaspoon ground cinnamon
1/2 teaspoon ground nutmeg
1 tablespoon honey or maple syrup (optional)
Salt and black pepper to taste
Fresh parsley for garnish (optional)

Instructions:

1. **Prepare the Sweet Potatoes:** Preheat your oven to 425°F (220°C). Peel and cut the sweet potatoes into 1-inch cubes.
2. **Season the Sweet Potatoes:** In a large bowl, toss the sweet potato cubes with olive oil, ground cinnamon, ground nutmeg, salt, and black pepper. If using, drizzle with honey or maple syrup for added sweetness.
3. **Roast the Sweet Potatoes:** Spread the seasoned sweet potatoes in a single layer on a baking sheet lined with parchment paper. Roast in the preheated oven for 25-30 minutes, or until the sweet potatoes are tender and caramelized, stirring halfway through for even cooking.
4. **Serve:** Remove from the oven and transfer to a serving dish. Garnish with fresh parsley if desired.

Nutrients (per serving)

Calories: 180 Sodium: 15 mg Carbohydrates: 32 g
Fiber: 5 g Protein: 2 g Calcium: 45 mg Fat: 7 g
Sugar: 8 g

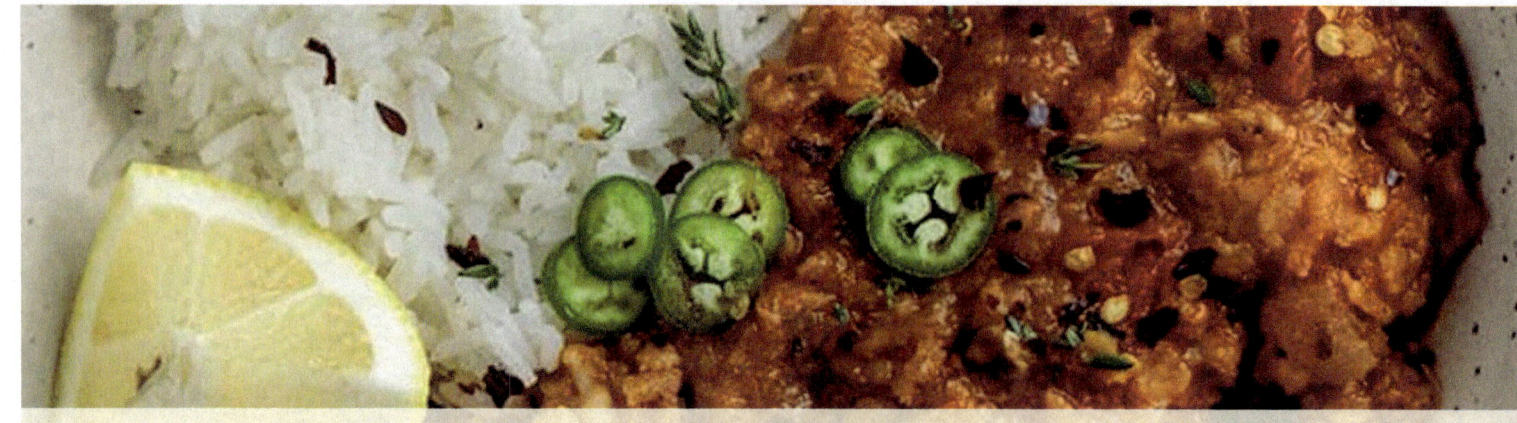

CAULIFLOWER AND LENTIL STEW

Cauliflower and Lentil Stew is a hearty and nutritious dish that combines the tender texture of cauliflower with protein-rich lentils. This stew is comforting, filling, and packed with vegetables, making it a perfect option for a wholesome meal.

Serves 	Preparation Time	Cooking Time 
4	15 minutes	35 minute

Ingredients:

1 tablespoon olive oil
1 onion, diced
2 garlic cloves, minced
1 carrot, diced
1 bell pepper, diced
1 head cauliflower, cut into florets
1 cup dried green or brown lentils, rinsed
1 can (14.5 oz) diced tomatoes
4 cups vegetable broth
1 teaspoon ground cumin
1 teaspoon paprika
1/2 teaspoon turmeric
1/2 teaspoon ground coriander
Salt and black pepper to taste
1 cup spinach or kale (optional)
Fresh cilantro for garnish (optional)

Instructions:

1. **Prepare the Vegetables:**
2. Dice the onion and carrot, mince the garlic, and dice the bell pepper. Cut the cauliflower into florets.
3. **Sauté the Aromatics:** Heat olive oil in a large pot over medium heat. Add the diced onion and cook for 4-5 minutes until it becomes translucent. Stir in the minced garlic and cook for an additional 1 minute until fragrant.
4. **Cook the Vegetables:** Add the diced carrot, bell pepper, and cauliflower florets to the pot. Sauté for 5-7 minutes until the vegetables start to soften.
5. **Add Lentils and Spices:** Stir in the rinsed lentils, diced tomatoes, vegetable broth, ground cumin, paprika, turmeric, and ground coriander. Season with salt and black pepper to taste.
6. **Simmer the Stew:** Bring the stew to a boil, then reduce the heat to low. Cover and simmer for 25-30 minutes, or until the lentils and vegetables are tender.
7. **Finish and Serve:** Stir in the spinach or kale if using, and cook for an additional 2-3 minutes until wilted. Garnish with fresh cilantro if desired.
8. **Serve:** Serve hot, either on its own or with a side of crusty bread or rice.

Nutrients (per serving)

Calories: 230 Sodium: 600 mg Carbohydrates: 37 g

Fiber: 12 g Protein: 12 g Calcium: 100 mg Fat: 6 g

Sugar: 7 g

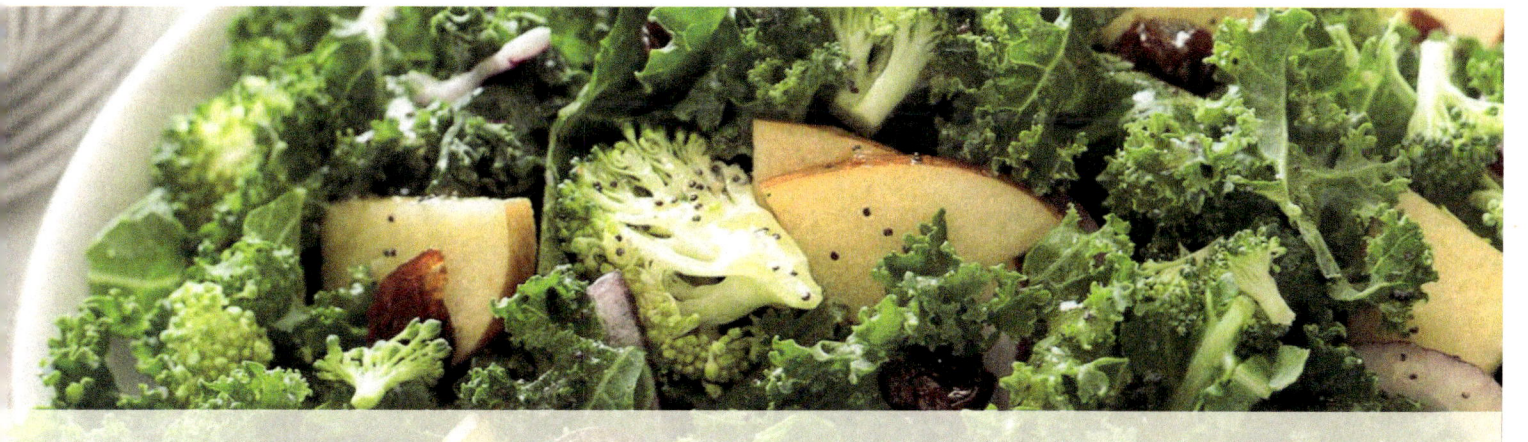

BROCCOLI AND KALE SALAD

Broccoli and Kale Salad is a vibrant and nutrient-packed dish that combines the crisp texture of broccoli with the hearty leaves of kale. Tossed in a light dressing and topped with crunchy almonds and tangy cranberries, this salad is both refreshing and satisfying.

Serves	Preparation Time	Cooking Time
4	10 minutes	0 minute

Ingredients:

2 cups fresh kale, stems removed and leaves chopped
2 cups broccoli florets, chopped
1/2 cup sliced almonds
1/4 cup dried cranberries
1/4 cup red onion, thinly sliced
1/4 cup feta cheese (optional)
1/4 cup olive oil
2 tablespoons apple cider vinegar
1 tablespoon honey or maple syrup
1 teaspoon Dijon mustard
Salt and black pepper to taste

Instructions:

1. **Prepare the Vegetables:** Wash and chop the kale leaves into bite-sized pieces. Cut the broccoli into small florets and lightly steam or blanch if desired for a more tender texture.
2. **Make the Dressing:** In a small bowl, whisk together olive oil, apple cider vinegar, honey or maple syrup, Dijon mustard, salt, and black pepper until well combined.
3. **Combine the Salad:** In a large salad bowl, combine the chopped kale, broccoli florets, sliced almonds, dried cranberries, and red onion. If using, add the feta cheese on top.
4. **Dress the Salad:** Drizzle the prepared dressing over the salad and toss gently until all the ingredients are evenly coated.
5. **Serve:** Serve immediately or chill in the refrigerator for 15-20 minutes to let the flavors meld.

Nutrients (per serving)

Calories: 220 Sodium: 150 mg Carbohydrates: 20 g
Fiber: 5 g Protein: 6 g Calcium: 100 mg Fat: 14 g
Sugar: 8 g

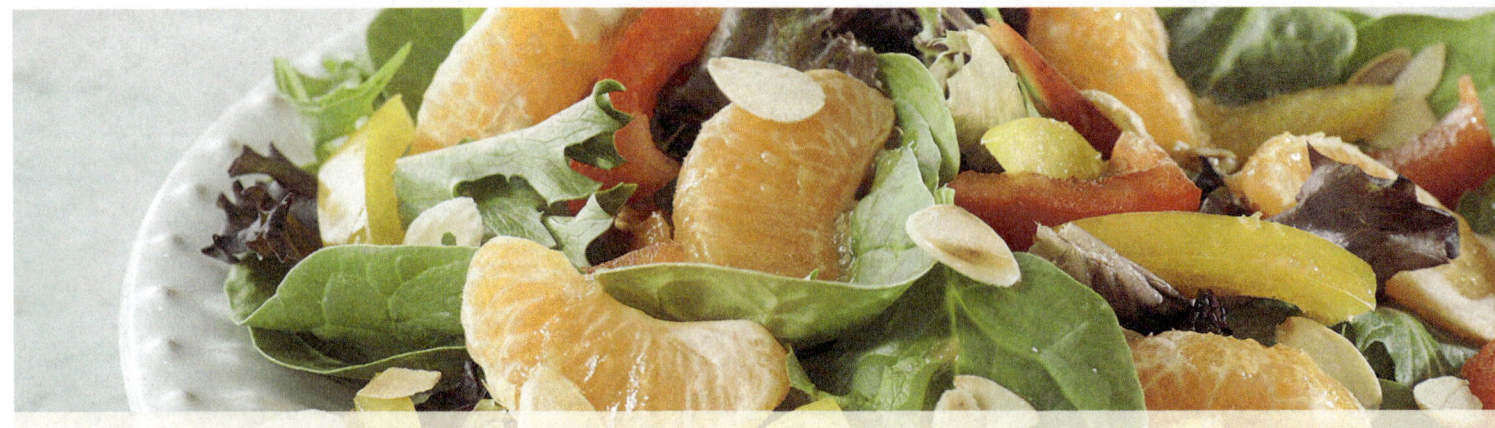

MIXED GREENS WITH CITRUS VINAIGRETTE

Mixed Greens with Citrus Vinaigrette is a refreshing and vibrant salad that features a variety of fresh greens topped with a zesty citrus dressing. It's a light and flavorful option that's perfect for a quick lunch or as a side dish.

Serves 	Preparation Time	Cooking Time 
4	10 minutes	0 minute

Ingredients:

4 cups mixed greens (such as arugula, spinach, and baby kale)
1/2 cup cherry tomatoes, halved
1/4 cup thinly sliced cucumber
1/4 cup red onion, thinly sliced
1/4 cup crumbled feta cheese (optional)
1/4 cup sliced almonds or walnuts (optional)

For the Citrus Vinaigrette:

1/4 cup freshly squeezed orange juice
2 tablespoons lemon juice
2 tablespoons olive oil
1 tablespoon honey or maple syrup
1 teaspoon Dijon mustard
Salt and black pepper to taste

Instructions:

1. Prepare the Salad Ingredients:
2. Wash and dry the mixed greens.
3. Halve the cherry tomatoes, slice the cucumber and red onion.
4. Make the Citrus Vinaigrette:
5. In a small bowl, whisk together orange juice, lemon juice, olive oil, honey or maple syrup, Dijon mustard, salt, and black pepper until well combined.
6. Combine the Salad:
7. In a large salad bowl, combine the mixed greens, cherry tomatoes, cucumber, and red onion.
8. If using, add the crumbled feta cheese and sliced almonds or walnuts.
9. Dress the Salad:
10. Drizzle the citrus vinaigrette over the salad and toss gently until all the ingredients are evenly coated.
11. Serve:
12. Serve immediately for the freshest taste, or chill in the refrigerator for 10-15 minutes to let the flavors blend.

Nutrients (per serving)

Calories: 180 Sodium: 150 mg Carbohydrates: 16 g
Fiber: 4 g Protein: 4 g Calcium: 100 mg Fat: 12 g
Sugar: 8 g

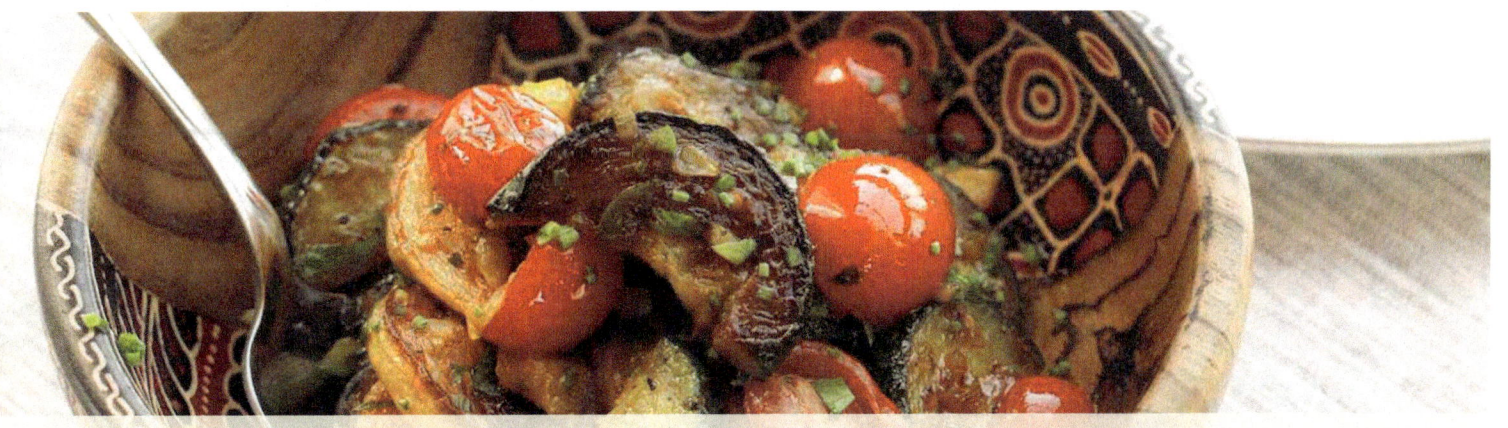

SAUTÉED ZUCCHINI WITH TOMATOES

Sautéed Zucchini with Tomatoes is a simple and delicious side dish that highlights the fresh flavors of zucchini and tomatoes. The dish is lightly seasoned and sautéed to create a tender, flavorful accompaniment that pairs well with a variety of main courses.

Serves 	Preparation Time	Cooking Time 
4	10 minutes	10 minute

Ingredients:

2 medium zucchinis, sliced into half-moons
1 cup cherry tomatoes, halved
2 tablespoons olive oil
2 garlic cloves, minced
1/2 teaspoon dried oregano
1/4 teaspoon dried basil
Salt and black pepper to taste
Fresh basil or parsley for garnish (optional)

w. Salmon / tuna steak.

Instructions:

1. **Prepare the Vegetables:** Slice the zucchinis into half-moons and halve the cherry tomatoes.
2. **Sauté the Garlic:** Heat olive oil in a large skillet over medium heat. Add minced garlic and sauté for 1 minute until fragrant, being careful not to let it burn.
3. **Cook the Zucchini:** Add the sliced zucchini to the skillet. Sauté for 5-7 minutes, or until the zucchini starts to soften and turn golden brown.
4. **Add Tomatoes and Seasonings:** Add the cherry tomatoes, dried oregano, dried basil, salt, and black pepper to the skillet. Continue to cook for an additional 3-4 minutes, or until the tomatoes are softened and the zucchini is tender.
5. **Serve:** Transfer the sautéed zucchini and tomatoes to a serving dish. Garnish with fresh basil or parsley if desired.

Nutrients (per serving)

Calories: 90 Sodium: 120 mg Carbohydrates: 10 g
Fiber: 3 g Protein: 2 g Calcium: 40 mg Fat: 6 g
Sugar: 4 g

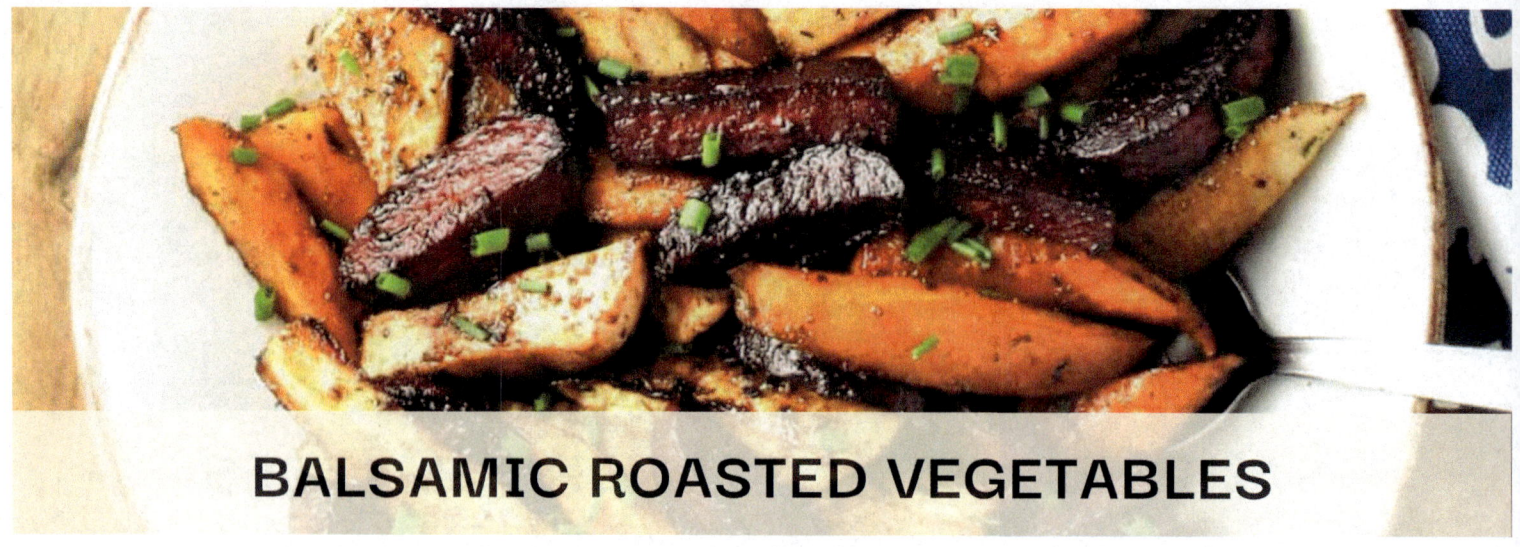

BALSAMIC ROASTED VEGETABLES

Balsamic Roasted Vegetables are a savory and tangy side dish that features a medley of vegetables roasted to perfection with a balsamic glaze. The balsamic vinegar enhances the natural sweetness of the vegetables, creating a deliciously caramelized flavor.

Serves 	Preparation Time	Cooking Time
4	15 minutes	25 minute

Ingredients:

1 cup carrots, peeled and cut into sticks
1 cup bell peppers, cut into chunks
1 cup zucchini, sliced
1 cup red onions, cut into wedges
2 tablespoons olive oil
2 tablespoons balsamic vinegar
1 tablespoon honey or maple syrup
1 teaspoon dried thyme
1 teaspoon dried rosemary
Salt and black pepper to taste
Fresh parsley for garnish (optional)

Instructions:

1. **Prepare the Vegetables:** Preheat your oven to 425°F (220°C).Peel and cut the carrots into sticks. Cut the bell peppers into chunks, slice the zucchini, and cut the red onions into wedges.
2. **Make the Balsamic Glaze:** In a small bowl, whisk together olive oil, balsamic vinegar, honey or maple syrup, dried thyme, dried rosemary, salt, and black pepper.
3. **Toss the Vegetables:** In a large mixing bowl, toss the prepared vegetables with the balsamic glaze until evenly coated.
4. **Roast the Vegetables:** Spread the vegetables in a single layer on a baking sheet.Roast in the preheated oven for 25-30 minutes, or until the vegetables are tender and caramelized, stirring halfway through.
5. **Serve:** Transfer the roasted vegetables to a serving dish.Garnish with fresh parsley if desired.

Nutrients (per serving)

Calories: 150 Sodium: 180 mg Carbohydrates: 20 g
Fiber: 5 g Protein: 2 g Calcium: 50 mg Fat: 8 g
Sugar: 10 g

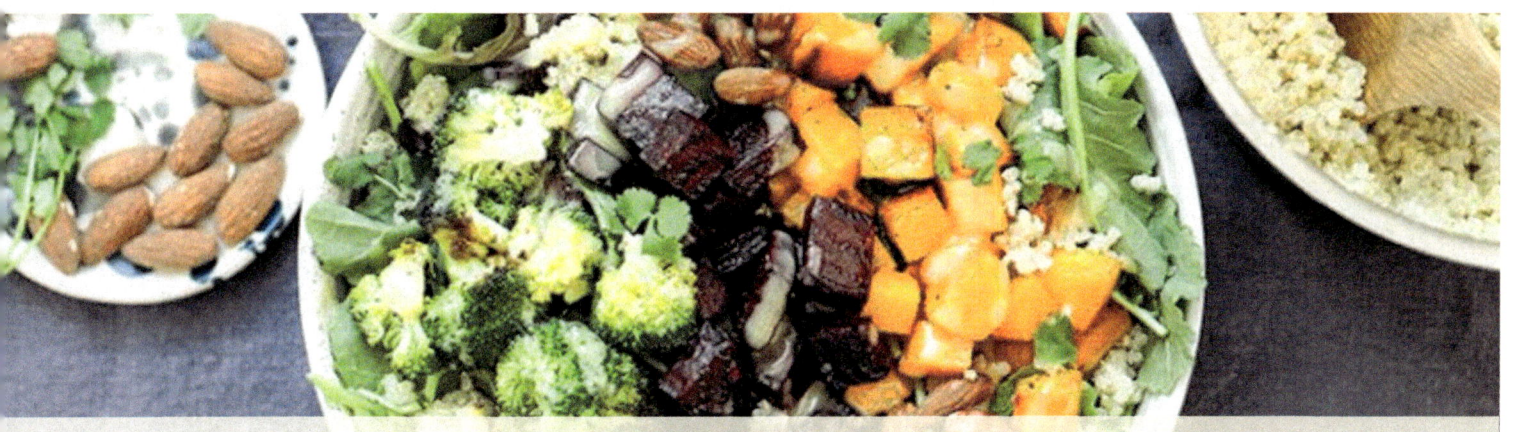

QUINOA AND ROASTED VEGETABLE BOWL

Quinoa and Roasted Vegetable Bowl is a nutritious and satisfying meal that combines protein-rich quinoa with a colorful assortment of roasted vegetables. Tossed with a light dressing and garnished with fresh herbs, it's perfect for a healthy lunch or dinner.

Serves	Preparation Time	Cooking Time
4	15 minutes	30 minute

Ingredients:

- 1 cup quinoa, rinsed
- 2 cups water or vegetable broth
- 1 cup bell peppers, cut into chunks
- 1 cup zucchini, sliced
- 1 cup cherry tomatoes, halved
- 1 cup red onions, cut into wedges
- 2 tablespoons olive oil
- 1 teaspoon dried oregano
- 1 teaspoon dried basil
- Salt and black pepper to taste
- 1/4 cup feta cheese (optional)
- Fresh parsley or basil for garnish (optional)

For the Dressing:
- 2 tablespoons olive oil
- 1 tablespoon lemon juice
- 1 teaspoon Dijon mustard
- 1 teaspoon honey or maple syrup
- Salt and black pepper to taste

Instructions:

1. **Cook the Quinoa:** In a medium saucepan, bring 2 cups of water or vegetable broth to a boil. Add the rinsed quinoa, reduce heat to low, cover, and simmer for 15 minutes, or until the quinoa is cooked and the liquid is absorbed. Fluff with a fork and set aside.
2. **Prepare the Vegetables:** Preheat your oven to 425°F (220°C). Cut the bell peppers, zucchini, cherry tomatoes, and red onions into appropriate sizes. Toss the vegetables with olive oil, dried oregano, dried basil, salt, and black pepper.
3. **Roast the Vegetables:** Spread the seasoned vegetables in a single layer on a baking sheet. Roast in the preheated oven for 20-25 minutes, or until the vegetables are tender and lightly caramelized, stirring halfway through.
4. **Make the Dressing:** In a small bowl, whisk together olive oil, lemon juice, Dijon mustard, honey or maple syrup, salt, and black pepper.
5. **Assemble the Bowl:** Divide the cooked quinoa among serving bowls. Top with the roasted vegetables. Drizzle with the prepared dressing. Sprinkle with feta cheese and garnish with fresh parsley or basil if desired.
6. **Serve:** Serve warm or at room temperature.

Nutrients (per serving)

Calories: 290 Sodium: 150 mg Carbohydrates: 40 g
Fiber: 7 g Protein: 10 g Calcium: 90 mg Fat: 10 g
Sugar: 8 g

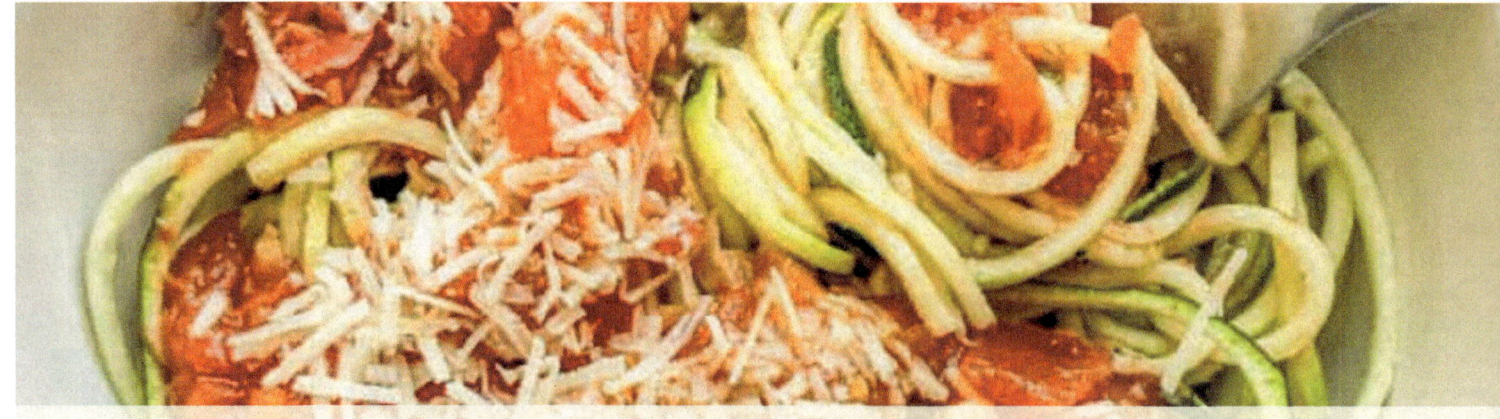

ZUCCHINI NOODLES WITH MARINARA SAUCE

Zucchini Noodles with Marinara Sauce is a light and satisfying dish that features spiralized zucchini as a healthy alternative to traditional pasta. Topped with a rich and flavorful marinara sauce, this dish is perfect for a low-carb, nutritious meal.

Serves 	Preparation Time	Cooking Time 
4	15 minutes	20 minute

Ingredients:

4 medium zucchinis, spiralized into noodles
2 tablespoons olive oil
1 onion, finely chopped
3 garlic cloves, minced
1 can (14.5 ounces) crushed tomatoes
2 tablespoons tomato paste
1 teaspoon dried oregano
1 teaspoon dried basil
1/4 teaspoon red pepper flakes (optional)
Salt and black pepper to taste
1/4 cup fresh basil, chopped (for garnish)
Grated Parmesan cheese (optional, for serving)

Instructions:

1. **Prepare the Zucchini Noodles:** Spiralize the zucchinis into noodles using a spiralizer or a vegetable peeler.
2. **Make the Marinara Sauce:** Heat olive oil in a large skillet over medium heat. Add the chopped onion and sauté until softened, about 5 minutes. Add the minced garlic and cook for an additional 1 minute. Stir in the crushed tomatoes, tomato paste, dried oregano, dried basil, red pepper flakes (if using), salt, and black pepper. Simmer the sauce for 10-15 minutes, stirring occasionally, until it thickens and the flavors meld together.
3. **Cook the Zucchini Noodles:** While the sauce is simmering, heat a separate skillet over medium heat. Add the zucchini noodles and cook for 2-3 minutes, stirring occasionally, until they are tender but still slightly crisp.
4. **Combine and Serve:** Toss the cooked zucchini noodles with the marinara sauce until well coated. Serve the zucchini noodles with marinara sauce in bowls. Garnish with chopped fresh basil and grated Parmesan cheese if desired.

Nutrients (per serving)

Calories: 130 Sodium: 250 mg Carbohydrates: 12 g
Fiber: 4 g Protein: 4 g Calcium: 80 mg Fat: 8 g
Sugar: 7 g

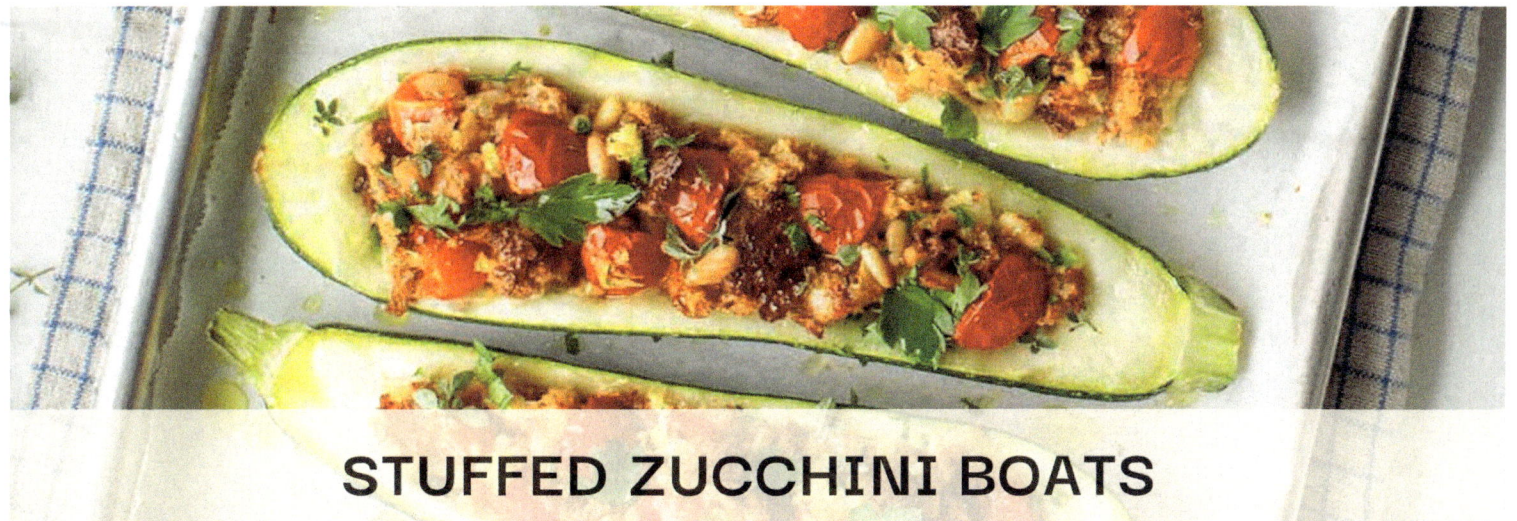

STUFFED ZUCCHINI BOATS

Stuffed Zucchini Boats are a versatile and delicious dish featuring zucchini halves filled with a savory mixture of ground meat, vegetables, and cheese. Baked until tender and topped with melted cheese, these boats make a satisfying main course or side dish.

Serves	Preparation Time	Cooking Time
4	15 minutes	25 minute

Ingredients:

4 medium zucchinis
1 tablespoon olive oil
1/2 pound ground turkey or beef   *chicken*
1/2 onion, finely chopped
2 garlic cloves, minced
1 cup diced tomatoes (canned or fresh)
1/2 cup cooked quinoa or rice (optional)
1/2 cup shredded mozzarella cheese
1/4 cup grated Parmesan cheese
1 teaspoon dried oregano
1 teaspoon dried basil
Salt and black pepper to taste
Fresh basil or parsley for garnish (optional)

Instructions:

1. **Prepare the Zucchini Boats:** Preheat your oven to 375°F (190°C). Slice the zucchinis in half lengthwise. Scoop out the seeds and some of the flesh to create boats, leaving a small border around the edges. Set aside.
2. **Cook the Filling:** Heat olive oil in a skillet over medium heat. Add the chopped onion and cook until softened, about 5 minutes. Add the minced garlic and cook for an additional 1 minute. Add the ground turkey or beef, cooking until browned and cooked through, breaking it up with a spoon. Stir in the diced tomatoes and cooked quinoa or rice (if using). Season with dried oregano, dried basil, salt, and black pepper. Simmer for 5 minutes to combine the flavors.
3. **Stuff the Zucchini Boats:** Place the zucchini halves on a baking sheet or in a baking dish. Spoon the meat mixture evenly into each zucchini boat. Sprinkle the shredded mozzarella cheese and grated Parmesan cheese on top of each stuffed zucchini.
4. **Bake the Zucchini Boats:** Bake in the preheated oven for 20-25 minutes, or until the zucchini is tender and the cheese is melted and bubbly.
5. **Serve:** Garnish with fresh basil or parsley if desired. Serve warm.

Nutrients (per serving)

Calories: 200 Sodium: 300 mg Carbohydrates: 12 g
Fiber: 4 g Protein: 20 g Calcium: 250 mg Fat: 10 g
Sugar: 6 g

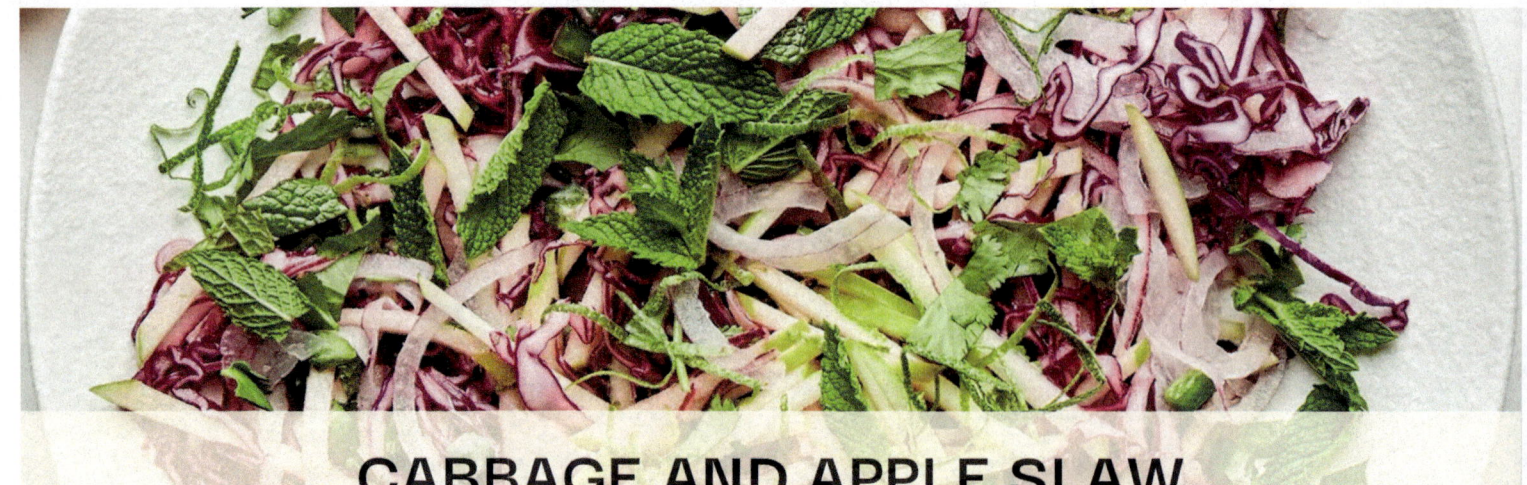

CABBAGE AND APPLE SLAW

Cabbage and Apple Slaw is a refreshing, crunchy side dish that pairs perfectly with a variety of meals. The crisp cabbage and sweet apples create a balanced flavor profile, making it a versatile and healthy addition to any table.

Serves	Preparation Time	Cooking Time
4	15 minutes	0 minute

Ingredients:

4 cups green cabbage, thinly sliced
1 cup red cabbage, thinly sliced
2 apples (Granny Smith or your favorite variety), julienned
1/2 cup shredded carrots
1/4 cup chopped fresh parsley
1/4 cup sliced green onions
1/3 cup mayonnaise (or Greek yogurt for a lighter option)
1 tablespoon ~~apple cider vinegar~~ *lemon juice*
1 tablespoon Dijon mustard
1 tablespoon honey or maple syrup
Salt and black pepper to taste

Instructions:

1. **Prepare the Vegetables:** In a large mixing bowl, combine the green and red cabbage, julienned apples, shredded carrots, chopped parsley, and sliced green onions.
2. **Make the Dressing:** In a small bowl, whisk together the mayonnaise, apple cider vinegar, Dijon mustard, honey (or maple syrup), salt, and black pepper until smooth.
3. **Toss the Slaw:** Pour the dressing over the cabbage and apple mixture. Toss well to evenly coat the vegetables with the dressing.
4. **Chill and Serve:** Cover the slaw and refrigerate for at least 30 minutes to allow the flavors to meld. Serve chilled as a side dish.

Nutrients (per serving)

Calories: 120 Sodium: 180 mg Carbohydrates: 15 g
Fiber: 4 g Protein: 2 g Calcium: 50 mg Fat: 7 g
Sugar: 10 g

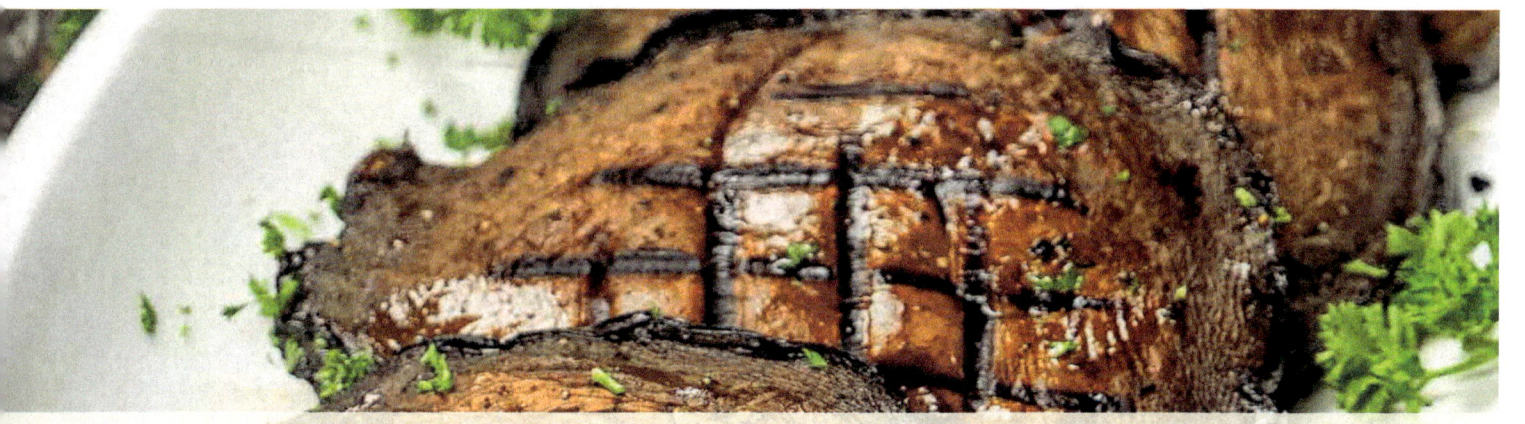

GRILLED PORTOBELLO MUSHROOMS

Grilled Portobello Mushrooms are a delicious and hearty dish, perfect as a vegetarian main course or a flavorful side. Their meaty texture and rich flavor make them a satisfying alternative to traditional grilled meats.

Serves	Preparation Time	Cooking Time
4	10 minutes	10 minute

Ingredients:

4 large Portobello mushrooms, stems removed
3 tablespoons olive oil
2 tablespoons balsamic vinegar
2 cloves garlic, minced
1 teaspoon dried thyme
1 teaspoon dried oregano
Salt and black pepper to taste
Fresh parsley for garnish (optional)

Instructions:

1. **Prepare the Marinade:** In a small bowl, whisk together the olive oil, balsamic vinegar, minced garlic, dried thyme, dried oregano, salt, and black pepper.
2. **Marinate the Mushrooms:** Place the Portobello mushrooms in a shallow dish or a resealable plastic bag. Pour the marinade over the mushrooms, ensuring they are well coated. Let them marinate for at least 20-30 minutes, turning occasionally to absorb the flavors.
3. **Grill the Mushrooms:** Preheat your grill to medium-high heat. Remove the mushrooms from the marinade and place them on the grill, gill side down. Cook for 4-5 minutes on each side, or until the mushrooms are tender and have grill marks.
4. **Serve:** Transfer the grilled mushrooms to a serving plate. Garnish with fresh parsley if desired. Serve immediately as a main dish or a side.

Nutrients (per serving)

Calories: 80 Sodium: 10 mg Carbohydrates: 6 g
Fiber: 2 g Protein: 2 g Calcium: 10 mg Fat: 6 g
Sugar: 2 g

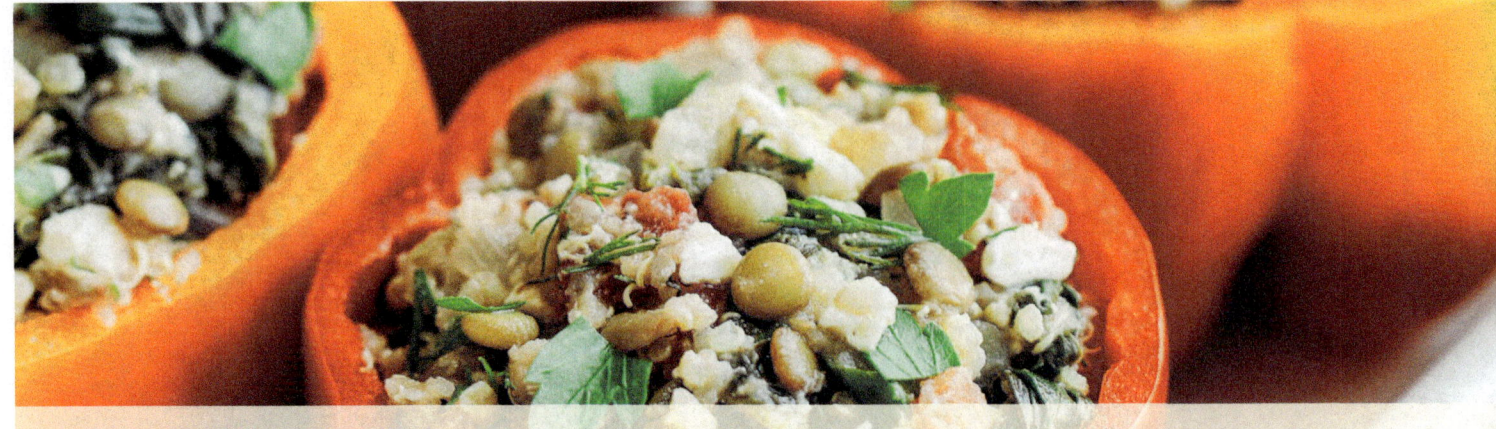

SPINACH AND QUINOA STUFFED PEPPERS

Spinach and Quinoa Stuffed Peppers are a healthy and flavorful dish, combining the nutty taste of quinoa with the vibrant freshness of spinach. These stuffed peppers are not only delicious but also packed with nutrients, making them an excellent option for a balanced meal.

Serves	Preparation Time	Cooking Time
4	20 minutes	45 minute

Ingredients:

4 large bell peppers (red, yellow, or green), tops cut off and seeds removed
1 cup quinoa, rinsed
2 cups vegetable broth or water
1 tablespoon olive oil
1 small onion, finely chopped
2 cloves garlic, minced
4 cups fresh spinach, chopped
1 teaspoon dried oregano
1 teaspoon dried basil
Salt and black pepper to taste
1/2 cup grated Parmesan cheese (optional)
1/4 cup chopped fresh parsley for garnish

Instructions:

1. **Prepare the Quinoa:** In a medium saucepan, bring the vegetable broth or water to a boil. Add the rinsed quinoa, reduce the heat to low, cover, and simmer for about 15 minutes or until the quinoa is cooked and the liquid is absorbed. Fluff the quinoa with a fork and set aside.
2. **Cook the Filling:** Heat olive oil in a large skillet over medium heat. Add the chopped onion and minced garlic, and sauté until the onion is soft and translucent, about 5 minutes. Add the chopped spinach to the skillet and cook until wilted, about 3-4 minutes. Stir in the cooked quinoa, dried oregano, dried basil, salt, and black pepper. Cook for an additional 2-3 minutes, mixing well to combine the flavors. If using, stir in the grated Parmesan cheese.
3. **Stuff the Peppers:** Preheat your oven to 375°F (190°C). Place the bell peppers in a baking dish. Spoon the quinoa and spinach mixture into each pepper, packing it in firmly.
4. **Bake the Peppers:** Cover the baking dish with aluminum foil and bake for 25-30 minutes, or until the peppers are tender. If desired, uncover the dish during the last 5 minutes to lightly brown the tops.
5. **Serve:** Remove the stuffed peppers from the oven and garnish with chopped fresh parsley. Serve hot as a satisfying main course.

Nutrients (per serving)

Calories: 200 Sodium: 300 mg Carbohydrates: 32 g
Fiber: 7 g Protein: 7 g Calcium: 100 mg Fat: 5 g
Sugar: 5 g

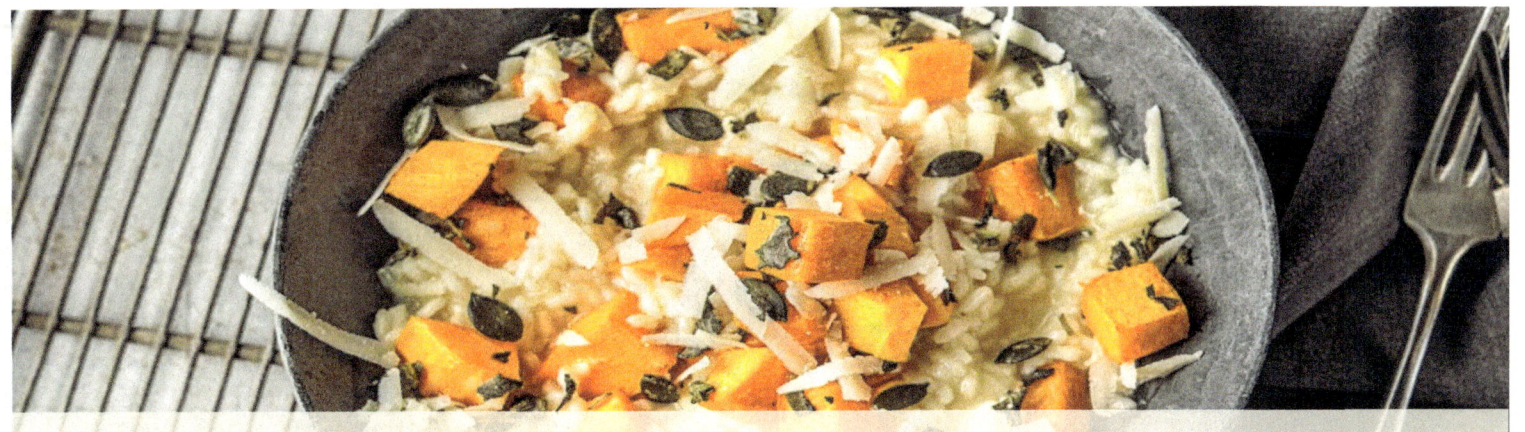

BUTTERNUT SQUASH AND SAGE RISOTTO

Butternut Squash and Sage Risotto is a comforting and creamy dish perfect for a cozy meal. The natural sweetness of roasted butternut squash pairs beautifully with the earthy aroma of fresh sage, creating a flavorful and satisfying risotto.

Serves	Preparation Time	Cooking Time 
4	15 minutes	45 minute

Ingredients:

1 small butternut squash, peeled, seeded, and diced into 1/2-inch cubes
2 tablespoons olive oil, divided
Salt and black pepper to taste
1 small onion, finely chopped
2 cloves garlic, minced
1 1/2 cups Arborio rice
1/2 cup dry white wine (optional)
4 cups vegetable broth, kept warm
1 tablespoon fresh sage, finely chopped
1/2 cup grated Parmesan cheese (optional)
2 tablespoons unsalted butter (optional)
Fresh sage leaves for garnish (optional)

Instructions:

1. **Roast the Butternut Squash:** Preheat your oven to 400°F (200°C). Toss the diced butternut squash with 1 tablespoon of olive oil, salt, and black pepper. Spread the squash in a single layer on a baking sheet and roast for 20-25 minutes, or until tender and lightly caramelized. Set aside.
2. **Cook the Risotto:** In a large, heavy-bottomed saucepan, heat the remaining tablespoon of olive oil over medium heat. Add the chopped onion and sauté until softened, about 5 minutes. Add the minced garlic and cook for another minute until fragrant. Stir in the Arborio rice and cook for 2-3 minutes, allowing the rice to toast slightly. If using, pour in the white wine and cook until it is mostly absorbed by the rice.
3. **Add the Broth:** Begin adding the warm vegetable broth to the rice, one ladleful at a time, stirring continuously. Allow the broth to be absorbed before adding more. Continue this process for about 18-20 minutes until the rice is creamy and al dente. You may not need all the broth.
4. **Finish the Risotto:** Stir in the roasted butternut squash and chopped fresh sage. If using, add the grated Parmesan cheese and butter, stirring until melted and well combined. Season with additional salt and black pepper to taste.
5. **Serve:** Spoon the risotto onto plates and garnish with fresh sage leaves if desired. Serve hot as a comforting main dish.

Nutrients (per serving)

Calories: 350 Sodium: 600 mg Carbohydrates: 60 g
Fiber: 4 g Protein: 8 g Calcium: 150 mg Fat: 8 g
Sugar: 4 g

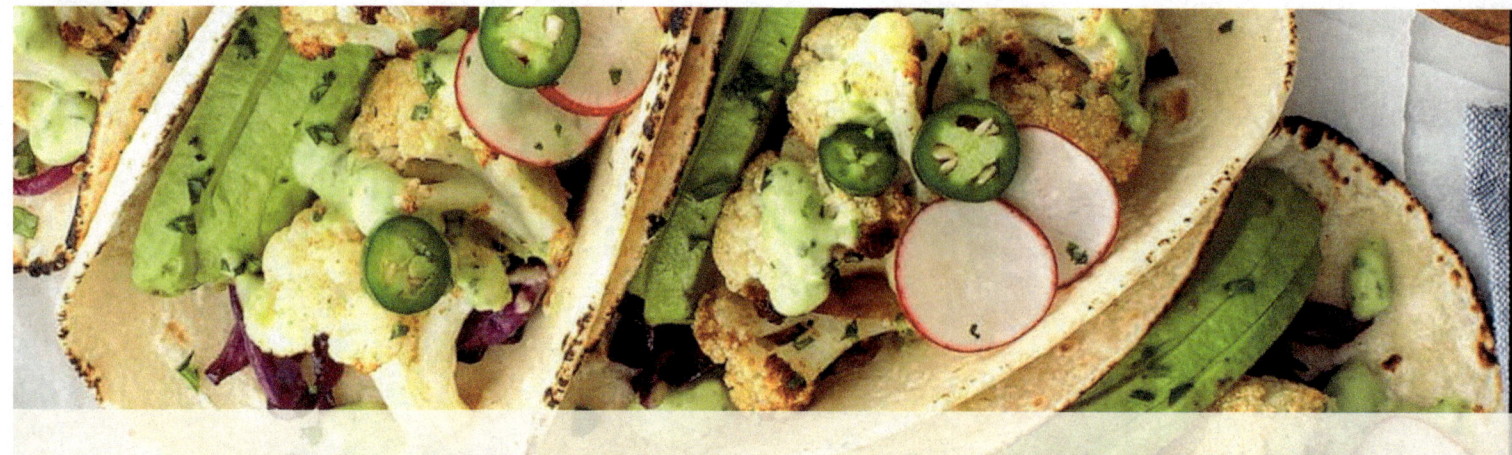

ROASTED CAULIFLOWER TACOS

Roasted Cauliflower Tacos are a vibrant and healthy twist on traditional tacos. Packed with flavor and texture, these tacos feature roasted cauliflower as the star ingredient, combined with fresh toppings and a zesty sauce.

Serves	Preparation Time	Cooking Time 
4	15 minutes	30 minute

Ingredients:

1 medium cauliflower, cut into small florets
2 tablespoons olive oil
1 teaspoon chili powder
1/2 teaspoon cumin
1/2 teaspoon smoked paprika
Salt and black pepper to taste
8 small corn tortillas
1/2 cup shredded red cabbage
1/2 cup diced tomatoes
1/4 cup chopped fresh cilantro
1 avocado, sliced
Lime wedges for serving

For the Sauce:
1/4 cup Greek yogurt
1 tablespoon lime juice
1/2 teaspoon hot sauce (optional)
Salt to taste

Instructions:

1. **Roast the Cauliflower:** Preheat your oven to 425°F (220°C). In a large mixing bowl, toss the cauliflower florets with olive oil, chili powder, cumin, smoked paprika, salt, and black pepper until well coated. Spread the cauliflower on a baking sheet in a single layer. Roast for 25-30 minutes, turning halfway through, until the cauliflower is golden brown and tender.
2. **Prepare the Sauce:** In a small bowl, whisk together the Greek yogurt, lime juice, hot sauce (if using), and a pinch of salt. Adjust seasoning to taste. Set aside.
3. **Assemble the Tacos:** Warm the corn tortillas in a dry skillet over medium heat or wrap them in foil and heat in the oven for a few minutes until pliable. Place a generous spoonful of roasted cauliflower onto each tortilla. Top with shredded red cabbage, diced tomatoes, sliced avocado, and fresh cilantro.
4. **Serve:** Drizzle the prepared yogurt sauce over the tacos and serve with lime wedges on the side for an extra burst of flavor.

Nutrients (per serving)

Calories: 250 Sodium: 400 mg Carbohydrates: 30 g
Fiber: 8 g Protein: 5 g Calcium: 60 mg Fat: 12 g
Sugar: 4 g

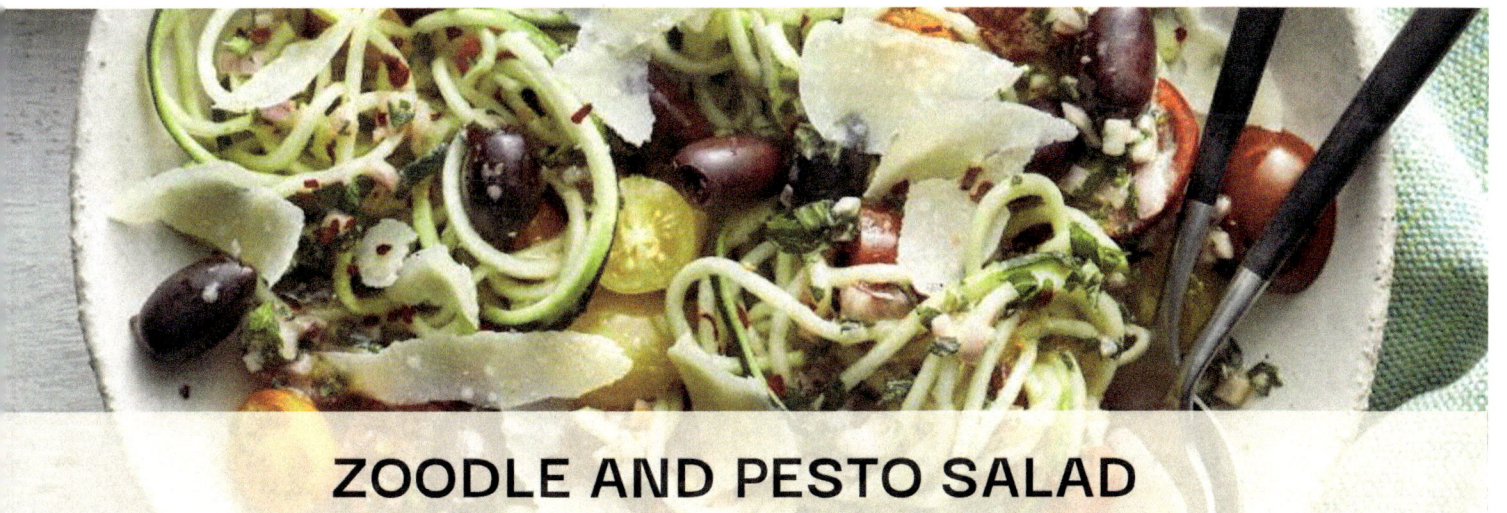

ZOODLE AND PESTO SALAD

Zoodle and Pesto Salad is a refreshing and low-carb dish featuring zucchini noodles tossed with a vibrant basil pesto. This salad is light, flavorful, and perfect for a quick lunch or side dish.

Serves	Preparation Time	Cooking Time 
4	15 minutes	0 minute

Ingredients:

2 medium zucchinis, spiralized into noodles (zoodles)
1/2 cup cherry tomatoes, halved
1/4 cup grated Parmesan cheese
1/4 cup toasted pine nuts
Salt and black pepper to taste
Fresh basil leaves for garnish

For the Pesto:
1 cup fresh basil leaves
1/4 cup olive oil
2 tablespoons grated Parmesan cheese
2 tablespoons pine nuts
1 garlic clove
Salt and black pepper to taste
Juice of 1/2 lemon

Instructions:

1. **Prepare the Pesto:** In a food processor, combine the fresh basil leaves, olive oil, Parmesan cheese, pine nuts, garlic, lemon juice, salt, and black pepper. Pulse until smooth, scraping down the sides as needed. Adjust seasoning to taste.
2. **Assemble the Salad:** In a large mixing bowl, toss the spiralized zucchini noodles with the prepared pesto until evenly coated. Add the cherry tomatoes, grated Parmesan, and toasted pine nuts to the bowl. Toss gently to combine all the ingredients.
3. **Serve:** Divide the zoodle salad into serving bowls. Garnish with fresh basil leaves and a sprinkle of black pepper. Serve immediately.

Nutrients (per serving)

Calories: 180 Sodium: 150 mg Carbohydrates: 7 g
Fiber: 2 g Protein: 5 g Calcium: 90 mg Fat: 15 g
Sugar: 3 g

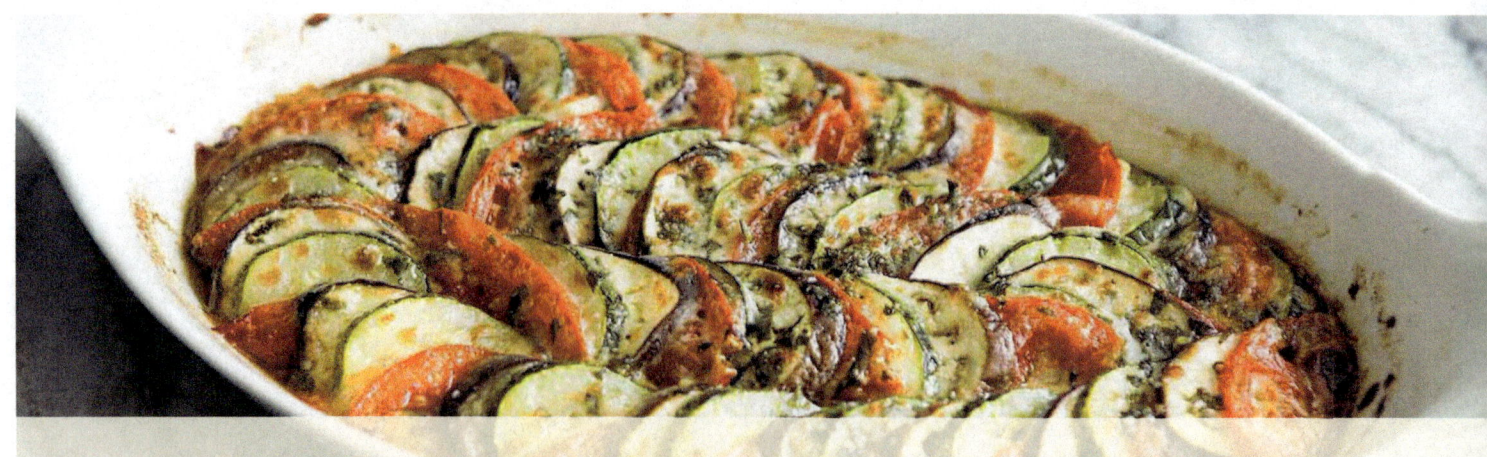

EGGPLANT AND TOMATO GRATIN

Eggplant and Tomato Gratin is a delicious, savory dish that layers tender eggplant and juicy tomatoes with a cheesy, herby topping. It's a great vegetarian option for dinner or a hearty side dish.

Serves	 Preparation Time	Cooking Time	
4	20 minutes	30 minute	

Ingredients:

2 medium eggplants, sliced into 1/4-inch rounds
4 medium tomatoes, sliced into 1/4-inch rounds
1 cup grated Parmesan cheese
1/2 cup grated mozzarella cheese
1/4 cup fresh basil leaves, chopped
2 tablespoons olive oil
2 garlic cloves, minced
Salt and black pepper to taste

Instructions:

1. **Prepare the Eggplant:** Preheat your oven to 375°F (190°C). Lay the eggplant slices on a baking sheet and sprinkle with salt. Let them sit for 15 minutes to draw out excess moisture. Pat them dry with a paper towel.
2. **Layer the Gratin:** In a large baking dish, arrange the eggplant slices in a single layer. Drizzle with olive oil and sprinkle with minced garlic. Place the tomato slices over the eggplant. Season with salt, black pepper, and chopped basil.
3. **Add Cheese and Bake:** Sprinkle the Parmesan and mozzarella cheese evenly over the top of the tomatoes and eggplant. Bake in the preheated oven for 25-30 minutes, or until the cheese is golden brown and bubbly, and the vegetables are tender.
4. **Serve:** Remove from the oven and let the gratin cool for a few minutes before serving. Garnish with additional fresh basil if desired.

Nutrients (per serving)

Calories: 210 Sodium: 300 mg Carbohydrates: 10 g
Fiber: 4 g Protein: 10 g Calcium: 180 mg Fat: 15 g
Sugar: 5 g

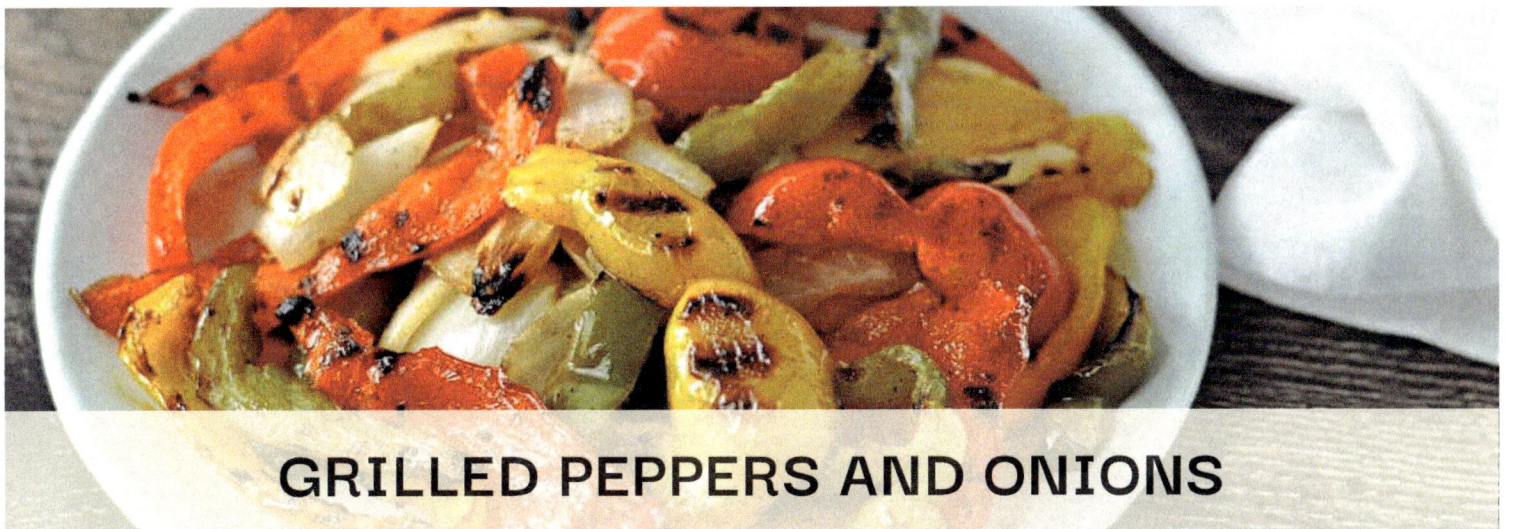

GRILLED PEPPERS AND ONIONS

Grilled Peppers and Onions is a simple, flavorful side dish perfect for pairing with your favorite protein or adding to sandwiches and wraps. The grilling brings out the natural sweetness of the vegetables, making them a delicious accompaniment to any meal.

Serves	Preparation Time	Cooking Time
4	10 minutes	10 minute

Ingredients:

2 large bell peppers (any color), sliced into strips
1 large red onion, sliced into rings
2 tablespoons olive oil
1 teaspoon balsamic vinegar
1 teaspoon dried oregano
Salt and black pepper to taste

Instructions:

1. **Prepare the Vegetables:** Preheat your grill to medium-high heat. In a large bowl, toss the bell pepper strips and onion rings with olive oil, balsamic vinegar, dried oregano, salt, and black pepper until evenly coated.
2. **Grill the Vegetables:** Place the pepper strips and onion rings directly on the grill grates. Grill for 8-10 minutes, turning occasionally, until the vegetables are tender and have a slight char.
3. **Serve:** Remove the peppers and onions from the grill and transfer them to a serving plate. Serve hot as a side dish or use them as toppings for sandwiches, tacos, or salads.

Nutrients (per serving)

Calories: 80 Sodium: 100 mg Carbohydrates: 8 g
Fiber: 2 g Protein: 1 g Calcium: 10 mg Fat: 5 g
Sugar: 4 g

DINNER

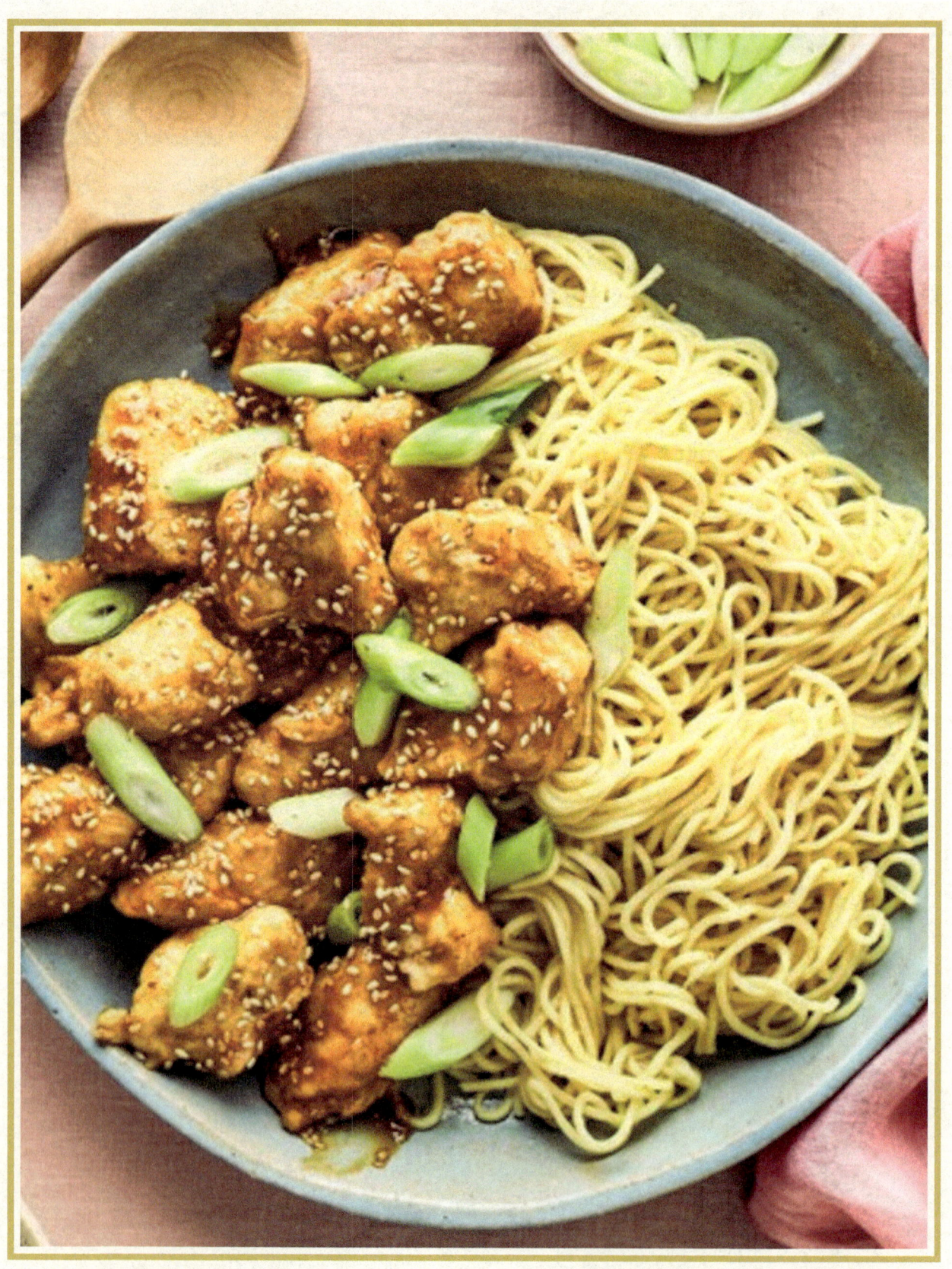

TABLE OF CONTENTS

- Grilled Lemon Herb Chicken (Yellow) — 78
- Salmon with Asparagus (Yellow) — 79
- Baked Salmon with Dijon Mustard (Yellow) — 80
- Beef and Broccoli Stir-Fry (Yellow) — 81
- Grilled Pork Tenderloin with Apples (Yellow) — 82
- Lemon Garlic Shrimp over Zoodles (Yellow) — 83
- Chicken and Broccoli Alfredo (with Zoodles) (Yellow) — 84
- Grilled Lamb Chops with Rosemary (Yellow) — 85
- Grilled Steak with Chimichurri Sauce (Yellow) — 86
- Chicken Caesar Salad (with Greek Yogurt Dressing) (Yellow) — 87
- Salmon and Quinoa Salad (Yellow) — 88
- Turkey and Spinach Stuffed Peppers (Yellow) — 89
- Chicken and Quinoa Stir-Fry (Yellow) — 90
- Tuna Salad Lettuce Wraps (Yellow) — 91
- Grilled Chicken with Avocado Salsa (Yellow) — 92
- Tuna and Avocado Salad (Yellow) — 93
- Chicken and Spinach Stuffed Mushrooms (Yellow) — 94
- Oven-Baked Chicken Tenders (Yellow)
- Baked Cod with Tomatoes and Olives (Yellow)

TABLE OF CONTENTS

- Turkey and Zucchini Burgers (Yellow) — 96
- Grilled Shrimp with Mango Salsa (Yellow) — 97
- Baked Chicken Parmesan (with Whole Wheat Breadcrumbs) (Yellow) — 98
- Turkey and Sweet Potato Hash (Yellow) — 99
- Turkey and Vegetable Meatloaf (Yellow) — 100
- Grilled Fish Tacos (Yellow) — 101
- Baked Chicken Thighs with Lemon (Yellow) — 102
- Turkey Meatballs with Zoodles (Yellow) — 103
- Honey Mustard Grilled Chicken (Yellow) — 104
- Garlic and Herb Grilled Pork Chops (Yellow) — 105
- Spicy Grilled Shrimp Skewers (Yellow) — 106
- Baked Salmon with Herbs (Yellow) — 107
- Balsamic Glazed Chicken (Yellow) — 108
- Turkey Stuffed Bell Peppers (Yellow) — 109
- Grilled Mahi Mahi with Pineapple Salsa (Yellow) — 110
- Baked Chicken Drumsticks (Yellow) — 111
- Lemon Butter Cod (Yellow) — 112
- Baked Tilapia with Lemon (Yellow) — 113
- Roasted Turkey Breast (Yellow) — 114

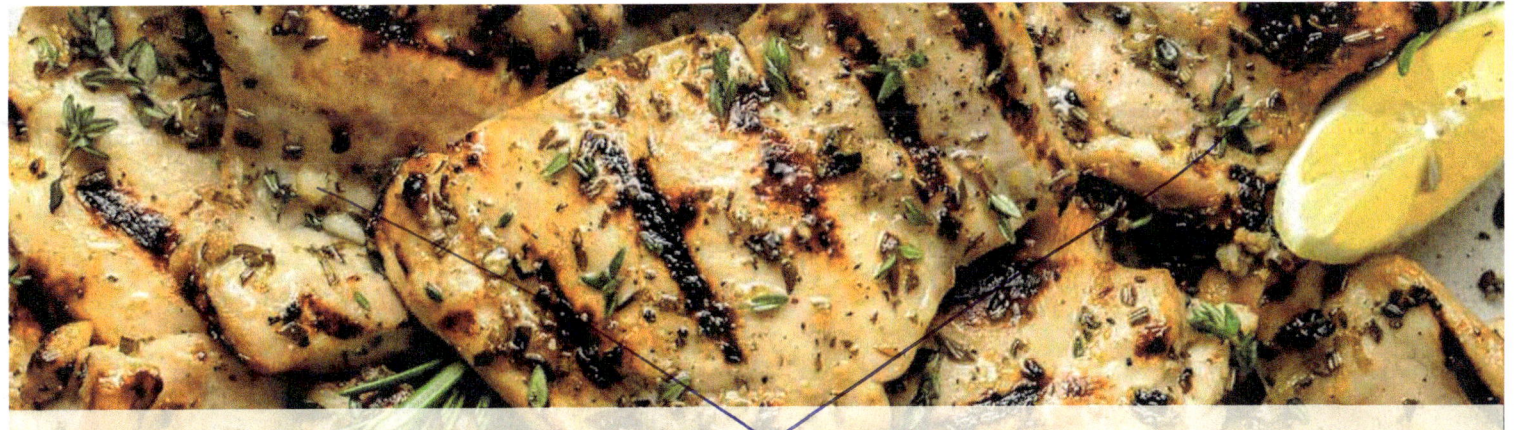

GRILLED PEPPERS AND ONIONS

Grilled Peppers and Onions is a simple, flavorful side dish perfect for pairing with your favorite protein or adding to sandwiches and wraps. The grilling brings out the natural sweetness of the vegetables, making them a delicious accompaniment to any meal.

Grilled chicken with lemon!

Serves	Preparation Time	Cooking Time
4	10 minutes	15 minute

Ingredients:

4 boneless, skinless chicken breasts — *THIN or butterfly*
3 tablespoons olive oil
Juice of 2 lemons
Zest of 1 lemon
3 garlic cloves, minced
1 tablespoon fresh rosemary, chopped
1 tablespoon fresh thyme, chopped
1 teaspoon dried oregano
Salt and black pepper to taste

or GRIDDLE

Instructions:

1. **Prepare the Marinade:** In a small bowl, whisk together olive oil, lemon juice, lemon zest, minced garlic, rosemary, thyme, oregano, salt, and black pepper.
2. **Marinate the Chicken:** Place the chicken breasts in a resealable plastic bag or a shallow dish. Pour the marinade over the chicken, ensuring all pieces are well-coated. Seal the bag or cover the dish and refrigerate for at least 30 minutes or up to 2 hours for the best flavor.
3. **Grill the Chicken:** Preheat your grill to medium-high heat. Remove the chicken from the marinade and shake off any excess. Grill the chicken for 6-8 minutes on each side, or until the internal temperature reaches 165°F (75°C) and the chicken is cooked through. *LONGER.*
4. **Serve:** Remove the chicken from the grill and let it rest for 5 minutes before serving. Serve the grilled lemon herb chicken with your favorite sides like grilled vegetables, salad, or quinoa.

w. salad new spuds

Nutrients (per serving)

Calories: 250 Sodium: 320 mg Carbohydrates: 2 g
Fiber: 0 g Protein: 32 g Calcium: 20 mg Fat: 12 g
Sugar: 0 g

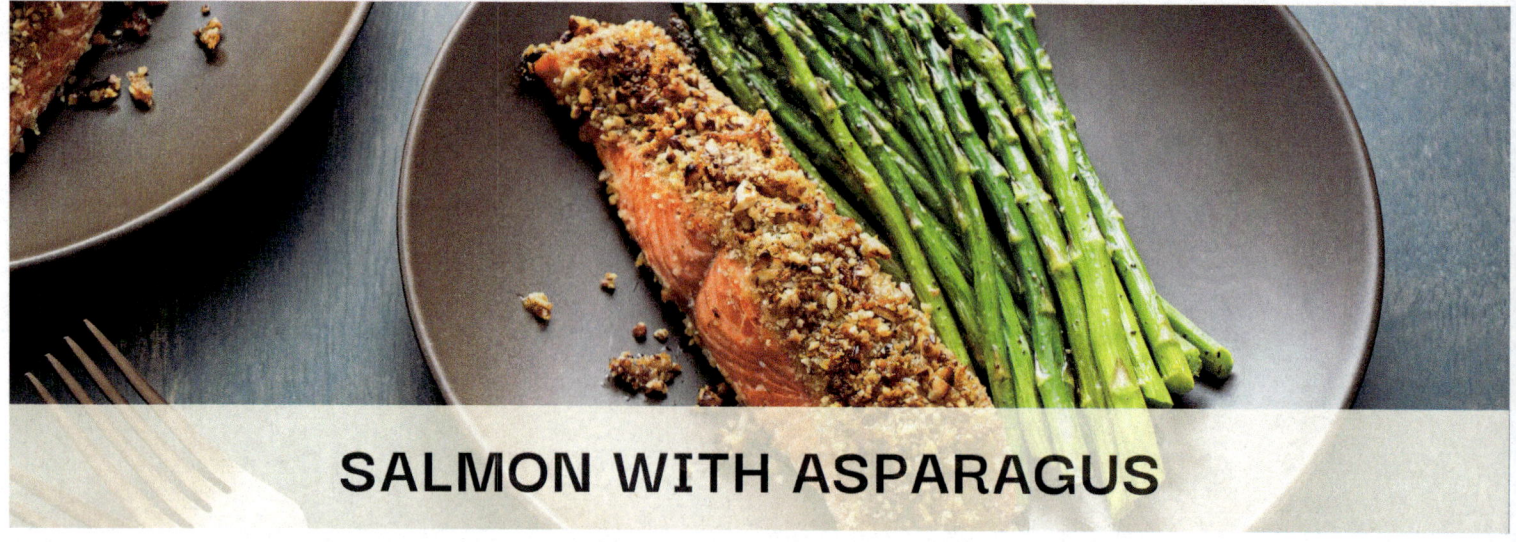

SALMON WITH ASPARAGUS

Salmon with Asparagus is a nutritious and elegant dish that's easy to prepare. The rich, buttery salmon pairs perfectly with the crisp-tender asparagus, making it a delightful meal for lunch or dinner.

Serves	Preparation Time	Cooking Time 
4	10 minutes	15 minute

Ingredients:

4 salmon fillets (about 6 oz each)
1 bunch asparagus, trimmed
2 tablespoons olive oil
2 cloves garlic, minced
Juice of 1 lemon
Zest of 1 lemon
1 tablespoon fresh dill, chopped (optional)
Salt and black pepper to taste

Instructions:

1. **Preheat the Oven:** Preheat your oven to 400°F (200°C).
2. **Prepare the Asparagus:** Arrange the trimmed asparagus on a baking sheet.Drizzle with 1 tablespoon of olive oil, and season with minced garlic, salt, and black pepper.Toss the asparagus to coat evenly.
3. **Prepare the Salmon:** Place the salmon fillets on top of the asparagus on the baking sheet.Drizzle the remaining olive oil over the salmon.Squeeze the lemon juice over the salmon and asparagus.Sprinkle lemon zest, dill (if using), salt, and black pepper over the top.
4. **Bake the Salmon and Asparagus:** Place the baking sheet in the preheated oven.Bake for 12-15 minutes, or until the salmon is cooked through and flakes easily with a fork, and the asparagus is tender.
5. **Serve:** Remove from the oven and let it rest for a minute before serving.Serve the salmon with asparagus, garnished with additional fresh dill and lemon wedges if desired.

Nutrients (per serving)

Calories: 300 Sodium: 250 mg Carbohydrates: 5 g
Fiber: 2 g Protein: 30 g Calcium: 50 mg Fat: 18 g
Sugar: 2 g

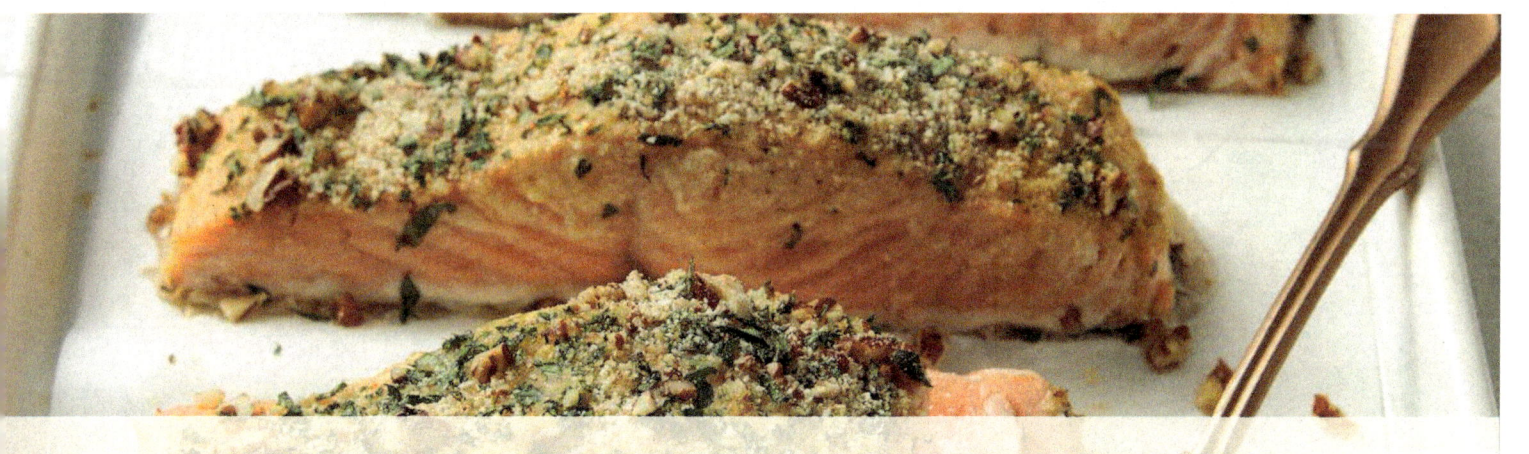

BAKED SALMON WITH DIJON MUSTARD

Baked Salmon with Dijon Mustard is a flavorful and easy-to-make dish that combines the rich taste of salmon with a tangy, savory Dijon mustard glaze. It's perfect for a quick weeknight dinner or a special occasion.

Serves 	Preparation Time	Cooking Time 
4	10 minutes	20 minute

Ingredients:

- 4 salmon fillets (about 6 oz each)
- 3 tablespoons Dijon mustard
- 2 tablespoons honey
- 1 tablespoon olive oil
- 1 tablespoon fresh lemon juice
- 2 cloves garlic, minced
- 1 teaspoon dried thyme or fresh thyme (chopped)
- Salt and black pepper to taste

Instructions:

1. **Preheat the Oven:** Preheat your oven to 375°F (190°C).
2. **Prepare the Glaze:** In a small bowl, whisk together Dijon mustard, honey, olive oil, lemon juice, minced garlic, thyme, salt, and black pepper until well combined.
3. **Prepare the Salmon:** Place the salmon fillets on a baking sheet lined with parchment paper or lightly greased. Brush each fillet generously with the Dijon mustard glaze.
4. **Bake the Salmon:** Place the baking sheet in the preheated oven. Bake for 15-20 minutes, or until the salmon is cooked through and flakes easily with a fork.
5. **Serve:** Remove the salmon from the oven and let it rest for a few minutes. Serve the baked salmon with your favorite side dishes, such as roasted vegetables, quinoa, or a fresh salad.

Nutrients (per serving)

Calories: 290 Sodium: 220 mg Carbohydrates: 10 g
Fiber: 1 g Protein: 30 g Calcium: 50 mg Fat: 16 g
Sugar: 8 g

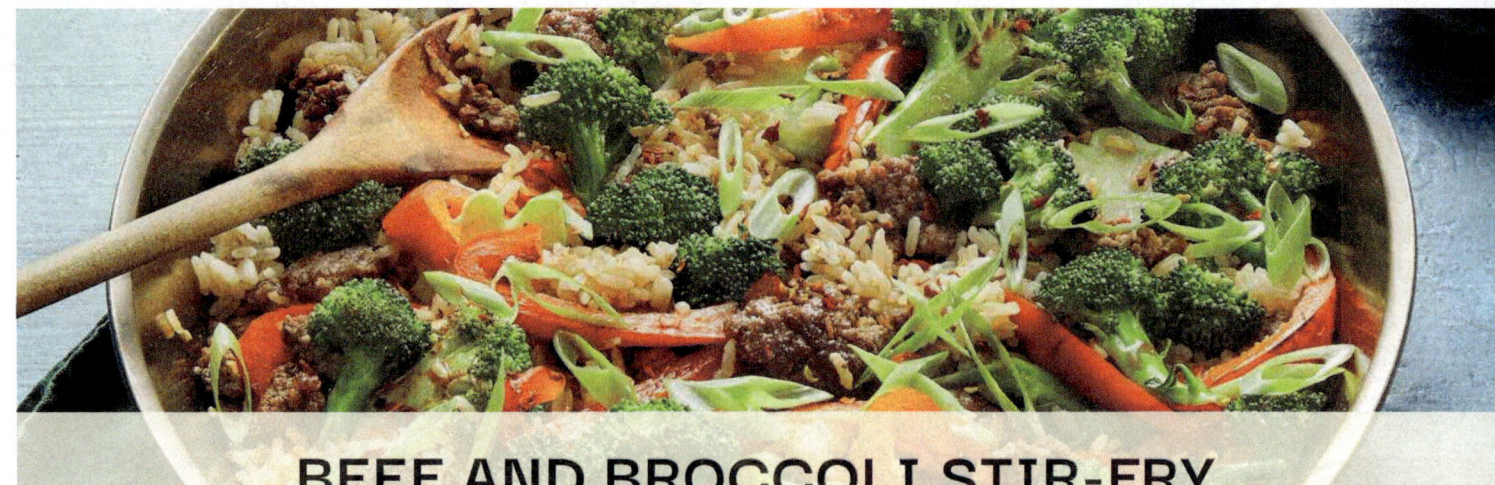

BEEF AND BROCCOLI STIR-FRY

Beef and Broccoli Stir-Fry is a classic Asian-inspired dish featuring tender beef slices and crisp broccoli florets, all tossed in a savory sauce. It's a quick and nutritious meal that's perfect for busy weeknights.

Serves	Preparation Time	Cooking Time
4	15 minutes	15 minute

Ingredients:

1 lb (450g) beef sirloin or flank steak, thinly sliced
3 cups broccoli florets
3 tablespoons soy sauce (low-sodium)
2 tablespoons oyster sauce
1 tablespoon hoisin sauce
1 tablespoon sesame oil
1 tablespoon cornstarch
1/2 cup beef broth or water
3 cloves garlic, minced
1-inch piece ginger, minced
2 tablespoons vegetable oil
1 tablespoon sesame seeds (optional)
Green onions, sliced (optional)
Salt and black pepper to taste

Instructions:

1. **Marinate the Beef:** In a bowl, combine the sliced beef with 1 tablespoon of soy sauce, 1 tablespoon of cornstarch, and a pinch of black pepper. Mix well and let it marinate for at least 10 minutes.
2. **Prepare the Sauce:** In a small bowl, whisk together the remaining soy sauce, oyster sauce, hoisin sauce, sesame oil, and beef broth or water. Set aside.
3. **Cook the Broccoli:** Heat 1 tablespoon of vegetable oil in a large skillet or wok over medium-high heat. Add the broccoli florets and stir-fry for 2-3 minutes until they are bright green and slightly tender. Remove the broccoli from the skillet and set aside.
4. **Cook the Beef:** In the same skillet, add the remaining tablespoon of vegetable oil. Add the minced garlic and ginger, and sauté for about 30 seconds until fragrant. Add the marinated beef to the skillet and stir-fry for 3-4 minutes until the beef is browned and cooked through.
5. **Combine and Serve:** Return the broccoli to the skillet with the beef. Pour the prepared sauce over the beef and broccoli, stirring to coat everything evenly. Cook for another 1-2 minutes until the sauce thickens slightly and the ingredients are heated through. Garnish with sesame seeds and sliced green onions, if desired. Serve hot with steamed rice or quinoa.

Nutrients (per serving)

Calories: 320 Sodium: 710 mg Carbohydrates: 12 g
Fiber: 3 g Protein: 28 g Calcium: 60 mg Fat: 18 g
Sugar: 4 g

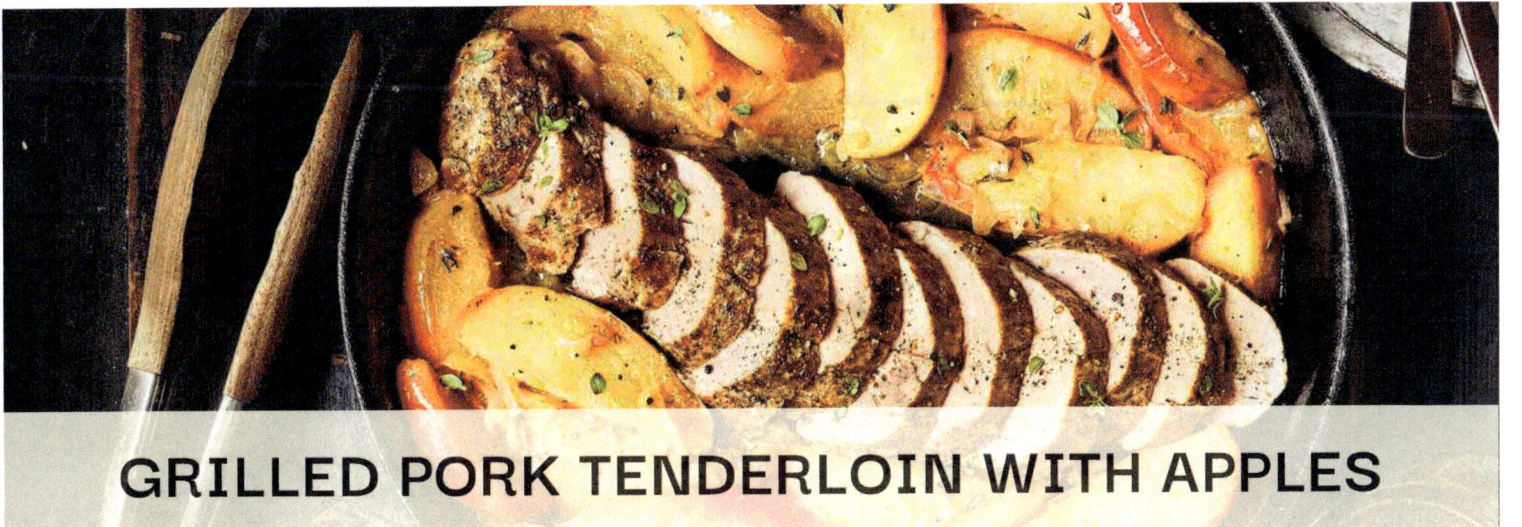

GRILLED PORK TENDERLOIN WITH APPLES

Grilled Pork Tenderloin with Apples is a delightful dish that combines the savory flavors of perfectly grilled pork with the sweet, tart taste of sautéed apples. It's an elegant yet simple meal, perfect for any occasion.

Serves 	Preparation Time	Cooking Time 
4	10 minutes	25 minute

Ingredients:

- 1 lb (450g) pork tenderloin
- 2 large apples, cored and sliced
- 1 tablespoon olive oil
- 2 tablespoons honey or maple syrup
- 1 teaspoon fresh rosemary, chopped
- 1 teaspoon fresh thyme, chopped
- 1/2 teaspoon ground cinnamon
- 1/4 teaspoon ground nutmeg
- Salt and black pepper to taste
- 1 tablespoon unsalted butter

Instructions:

1. **Prepare the Pork Tenderloin:** Preheat your grill to medium-high heat. Rub the pork tenderloin with olive oil, and season it generously with salt, black pepper, rosemary, and thyme.
2. **Grill the Pork Tenderloin:** Place the pork tenderloin on the preheated grill. Grill the pork for about 15-20 minutes, turning occasionally, until it reaches an internal temperature of 145°F (63°C). Once cooked, remove the pork from the grill and let it rest for 5 minutes before slicing.
3. **Cook the Apples:** While the pork is grilling, melt the butter in a large skillet over medium heat. Add the apple slices to the skillet and sprinkle with cinnamon and nutmeg. Drizzle the honey or maple syrup over the apples and stir to combine. Sauté the apples for about 5-7 minutes, until they are soft and slightly caramelized.
4. **Serve:** Slice the grilled pork tenderloin into medallions. Arrange the pork slices on a serving platter and top with the sautéed apples. Garnish with extra fresh rosemary or thyme if desired, and serve immediately.

Nutrients (per serving)

Calories: 320 Sodium: 140 mg Carbohydrates: 22 g

Fiber: 3 g Protein: 24 g Calcium: 30 mg Fat: 12 g

Sugar: 18 g

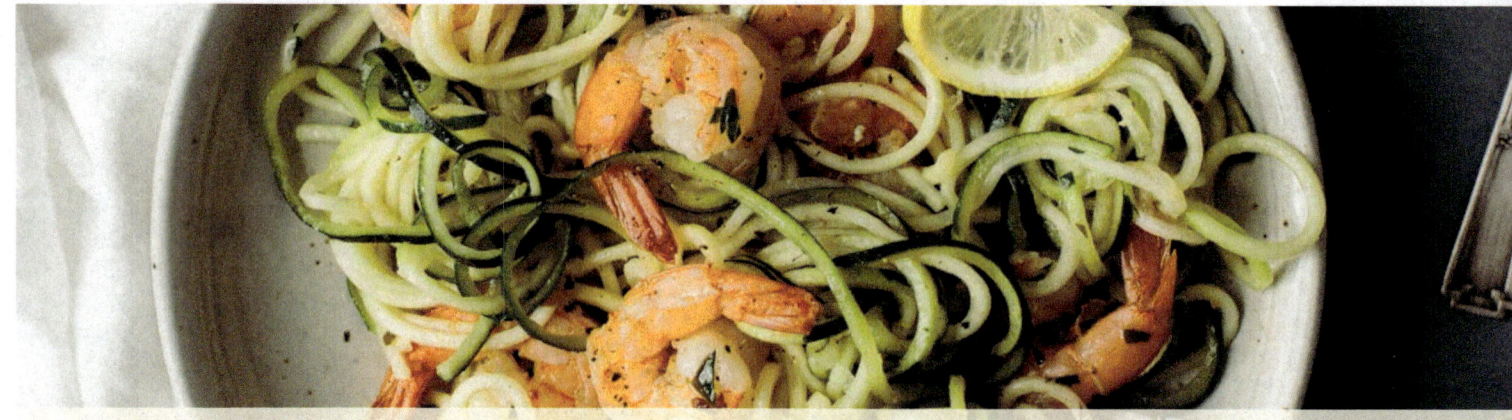

LEMON GARLIC SHRIMP OVER ZOODLES

Lemon Garlic Shrimp over Zoodles is a light and flavorful dish that pairs tender shrimp with zucchini noodles for a healthy, low-carb meal. The bright lemon and garlic flavors make it a refreshing option for any time of the year.

Serves	Preparation Time	Cooking Time 
4	10 minutes	10 minute

Ingredients:

1 lb (450g) shrimp, peeled and deveined
4 medium zucchinis, spiralized into noodles
2 tablespoons olive oil
3 cloves garlic, minced
1 lemon, zested and juiced
1/4 teaspoon red pepper flakes (optional)
Salt and black pepper to taste
2 tablespoons fresh parsley, chopped
1/4 cup grated Parmesan cheese (optional)

Instructions:

1. **Prepare the Shrimp:** In a large skillet, heat 1 tablespoon of olive oil over medium heat.Add the minced garlic and red pepper flakes (if using) to the skillet, and sauté for 1-2 minutes until fragrant.Add the shrimp to the skillet, seasoning with salt, black pepper, and lemon zest.Cook the shrimp for 2-3 minutes on each side until they are pink and fully cooked. Remove the shrimp from the skillet and set aside.
2. **Cook the Zoodles:** In the same skillet, add the remaining tablespoon of olive oil.Add the spiralized zucchini noodles to the skillet, and sauté for 2-3 minutes until they are just tender but still slightly crisp.Season the zoodles with salt, black pepper, and lemon juice.
3. **Assemble the Dish:** Add the cooked shrimp back to the skillet with the zoodles.Toss everything together to combine, ensuring the shrimp is well distributed among the zoodles.Sprinkle with fresh parsley and grated Parmesan cheese if desired.
4. **Serve:** Divide the Lemon Garlic Shrimp over Zoodles among serving plates.Serve immediately, garnished with additional lemon wedges or parsley if desired.

Nutrients (per serving)

Calories: 210 Sodium: 410 mg Carbohydrates: 8 g
Fiber: 2 g Protein: 26 g Calcium: 110 mg Fat: 10 g
Sugar: 4 g

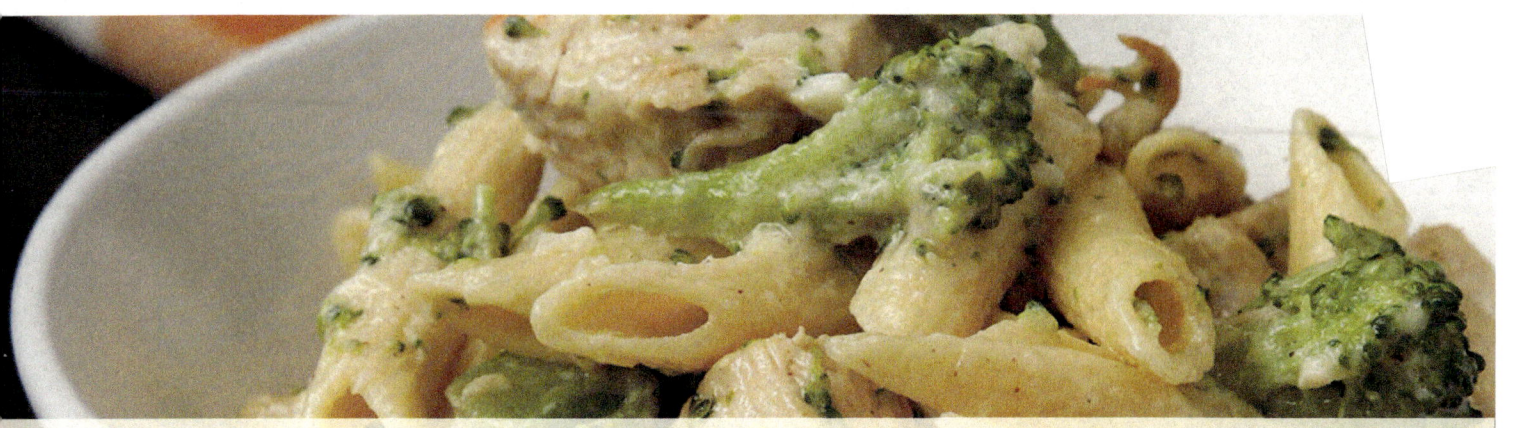

CHICKEN AND BROCCOLI ALFREDO

Chicken and Broccoli Alfredo with Zoodles is a creamy, low-carb twist on the classic Alfredo pasta. By swapping out traditional pasta for zucchini noodles, this dish remains rich and satisfying while being lighter and packed with nutrients.

Serves	Preparation Time	Cooking Time
4	15 minutes	15 minute

Ingredients:

- 2 large chicken breasts, sliced into thin strips
- 4 medium zucchinis, spiralized into noodles
- 2 cups broccoli florets
- 1 tablespoon olive oil
- 3 cloves garlic, minced
- 1/2 cup heavy cream
- 1/2 cup grated Parmesan cheese
- 1/4 cup cream cheese
- 1/2 teaspoon garlic powder
- Salt and black pepper to taste
- Fresh parsley, chopped (for garnish)
- Optional: Red pepper flakes for a bit of heat

Instructions:

1. **Cook the Chicken:** Heat olive oil in a large skillet over medium heat. Add the sliced chicken breasts to the skillet, seasoning with salt, black pepper, and garlic powder. Cook the chicken for 6-7 minutes, or until fully cooked and slightly browned. Remove from the skillet and set aside.
2. **Cook the Broccoli:** In the same skillet, add the broccoli florets and cook for 3-4 minutes until they are tender but still crisp. Set the broccoli aside with the chicken.
3. **Prepare the Alfredo Sauce:** In the same skillet, add the minced garlic and sauté for about 1 minute until fragrant. Reduce the heat to low, then add the heavy cream and cream cheese to the skillet. Stir continuously until the cream cheese has melted and the sauce is smooth. Gradually stir in the grated Parmesan cheese, allowing it to melt into the sauce. Season the sauce with additional salt, black pepper, and red pepper flakes if desired.
4. **Cook the Zoodles:** Add the spiralized zucchini noodles to the skillet with the Alfredo sauce. Toss the zoodles in the sauce for 2-3 minutes until they are slightly tender but still have some crunch.
5. **Assemble the Dish:** Add the cooked chicken and broccoli back into the skillet with the zoodles and sauce. Toss everything together to ensure the chicken, broccoli, and zoodles are well-coated in the Alfredo sauce.
6. **Serve:** Divide the Chicken and Broccoli Alfredo with Zoodles among serving plates. Garnish with chopped parsley and additional Parmesan cheese if desired.

Nutrients (per serving)

Calories: 350 Sodium: 520 mg Carbohydrates: 9 g

Fiber: 3 g Protein: 32 g Calcium: 220 mg Fat: 22 g

Sugar: 5 g

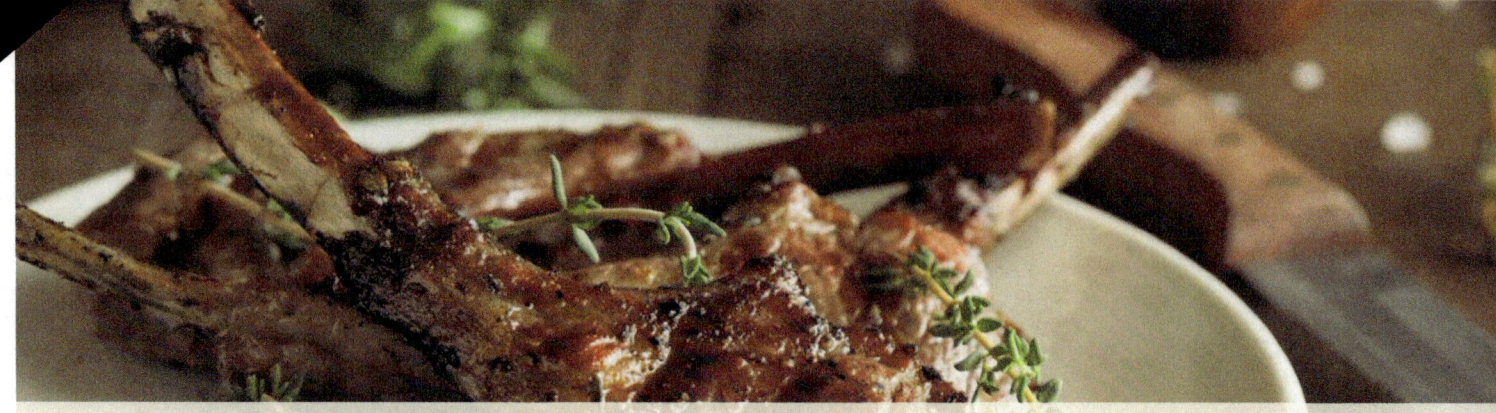

GRILLED LAMB CHOPS WITH ROSEMARY

Grilled Lamb Chops with Rosemary is a classic and flavorful dish that highlights the rich taste of lamb, enhanced by the aromatic infusion of fresh rosemary. This simple yet elegant meal is perfect for special occasions or a sophisticated dinner at home.

Serves 	Preparation Time	Cooking Time 
4	10 minutes	8 minute

Ingredients:

- 8 lamb chops
- 2 tablespoons fresh rosemary, finely chopped
- 3 cloves garlic, minced
- 2 tablespoons olive oil
- 1 tablespoon lemon juice
- Salt and black pepper to taste
- Optional: Lemon wedges for serving

Instructions:

1. **Prepare the Marinade:** In a small bowl, combine the chopped rosemary, minced garlic, olive oil, lemon juice, salt, and black pepper. Mix well to create a fragrant marinade.
2. **Marinate the Lamb Chops:** Place the lamb chops in a large dish or resealable plastic bag. Pour the rosemary marinade over the lamb chops, ensuring each chop is evenly coated. Cover the dish or seal the bag and let the lamb chops marinate in the refrigerator for at least 30 minutes, or up to 4 hours for more intense flavor.
3. **Preheat the Grill:** Preheat your grill to medium-high heat. Make sure the grates are clean and lightly oiled to prevent sticking.
4. **Grill the Lamb Chops:** Remove the lamb chops from the marinade, allowing any excess to drip off. Place the lamb chops on the preheated grill. Grill the lamb chops for about 3-4 minutes per side for medium-rare, or longer if you prefer your lamb more well-done. Use tongs to flip the chops, ensuring they are evenly cooked and have nice grill marks.
5. **Rest and Serve:** Once the lamb chops are grilled to your desired doneness, remove them from the grill. Let the lamb chops rest for 5 minutes to allow the juices to redistribute. Serve the grilled lamb chops with optional lemon wedges on the side for an extra burst of citrus flavor.

Nutrients (per serving)

Calories: 320 Sodium: 340 mg Carbohydrates: 1 g
Fiber: 0 g Protein: 28 g Calcium: 30 mg Fat: 22 g
Sugar: 0 g

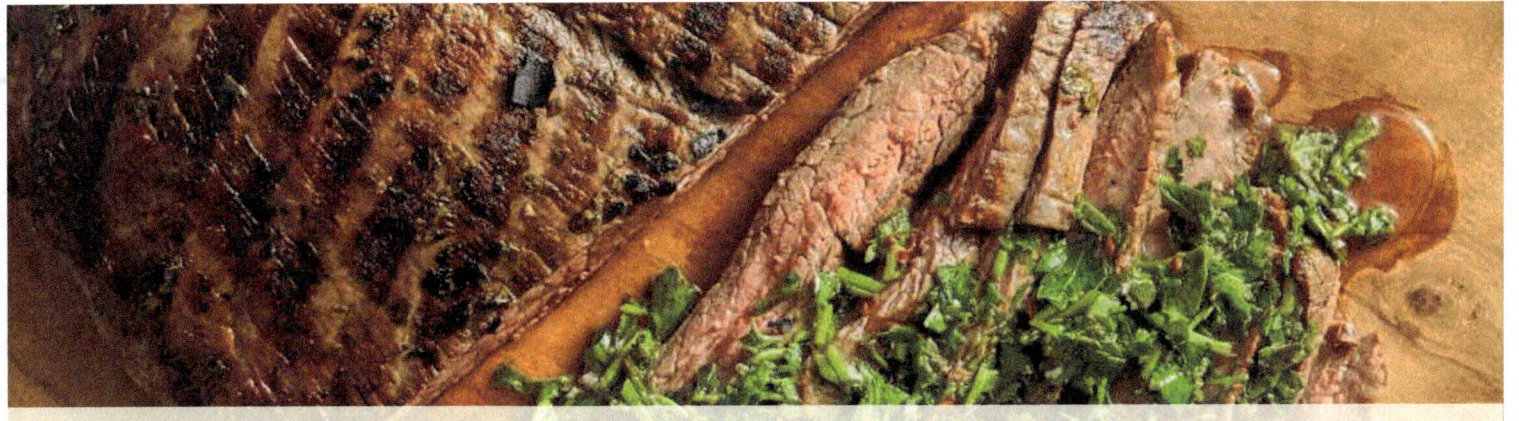

GRILLED STEAK WITH CHIMICHURRI SAUCE

Grilled Steak with Chimichurri Sauce is a vibrant and flavorful dish that brings together the juicy tenderness of a perfectly grilled steak with the fresh, tangy flavors of a classic chimichurri sauce. This dish is a favorite for barbecues and outdoor dining, offering a delicious balance of savory meat and herbaceous sauce.

Serves 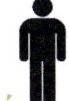	Preparation Time	Cooking Time
4	10 minutes	10 minute

Ingredients:

4 ribeye or sirloin steaks (about 1-inch thick)
2 tablespoons olive oil
Salt and black pepper to taste
For the Chimichurri Sauce:
1 cup fresh parsley, finely chopped
1/4 cup fresh cilantro, finely chopped (optional)
4 cloves garlic, minced
2 tablespoons red wine vinegar
1/2 teaspoon red pepper flakes
1/2 cup olive oil
Salt and black pepper to taste

Instructions:

1. **Prepare the Chimichurri Sauce:** In a medium bowl, combine the chopped parsley, cilantro (if using), minced garlic, red wine vinegar, and red pepper flakes.Slowly whisk in the olive oil until the sauce is well combined.Season with salt and black pepper to taste.Set the chimichurri sauce aside to allow the flavors to meld while you prepare the steak.
2. **Preheat the Grill:** Preheat your grill to high heat. Ensure the grates are clean and lightly oiled to prevent sticking.
3. **Season the Steaks:** Rub the steaks with olive oil on both sides.Generously season the steaks with salt and black pepper.
4. **Grill the Steaks:** Place the steaks on the preheated grill.Grill the steaks for about 4-5 minutes per side for medium-rare, or adjust the time according to your preferred level of doneness.Use tongs to flip the steaks, ensuring they get a nice sear on both sides.
5. **Rest the Steaks:** Once the steaks are grilled to your desired doneness, remove them from the grill.Let the steaks rest for 5 minutes to allow the juices to redistribute.
6. **Serve:** Slice the grilled steaks against the grain for maximum tenderness.Spoon the chimichurri sauce generously over the steak slices before serving.Serve with your favorite sides for a complete meal.

Nutrients (per serving)

Calories: 450 Sodium: 400 mg Carbohydrates: 2 g
Fiber: 1 g Protein: 35 g Calcium: 40 mg Fat: 34 g
Sugar: 0 g

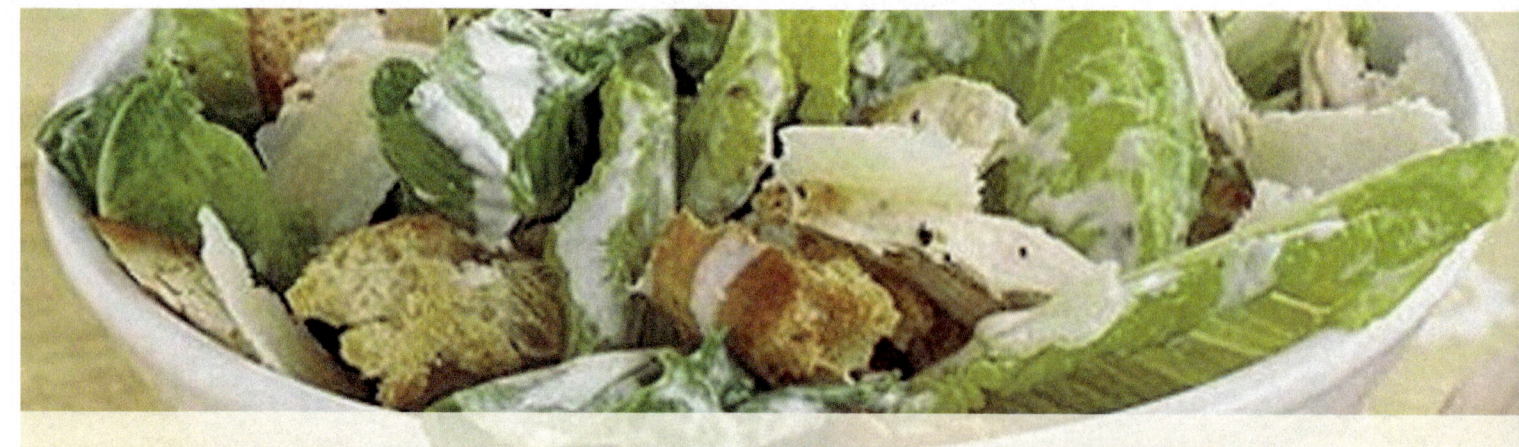

CHICKEN CAESAR SALAD

Chicken Caesar Salad is a classic dish that combines crisp romaine lettuce, juicy grilled chicken, crunchy croutons, and a rich, creamy Caesar dressing. It's a hearty salad that's both satisfying and refreshing, perfect for a light lunch or dinner.

Serves 	Preparation Time	Cooking Time
4	10 minutes	15 minute

Ingredients:

2 boneless, skinless chicken breasts
1 tablespoon olive oil
Salt and black pepper to taste
1 large head of romaine lettuce, chopped
1/2 cup Caesar dressing
1/4 cup grated Parmesan cheese
1 cup croutons
1 lemon, cut into wedges (optional)

Instructions:

1. **Prepare the Chicken:** Preheat a grill or grill pan over medium-high heat. Rub the chicken breasts with olive oil and season with salt and black pepper on both sides. Grill the chicken for 6-7 minutes on each side, or until fully cooked and the internal temperature reaches 165°F (74°C). Remove the chicken from the grill and let it rest for a few minutes before slicing it into thin strips.
2. **Assemble the Salad:** In a large salad bowl, combine the chopped romaine lettuce, Caesar dressing, and grated Parmesan cheese. Toss the salad until the lettuce is evenly coated with the dressing.
3. **Add the Chicken and Croutons:** Top the salad with the sliced grilled chicken and croutons. Give the salad a final toss to distribute the chicken and croutons evenly.
4. **Serve:** Divide the salad into serving bowls. Garnish with additional Parmesan cheese and a squeeze of lemon juice if desired. Serve immediately for the best flavor and texture.

Nutrients (per serving)

Calories: 350 Sodium: 800 mg Carbohydrates: 10 g
Fiber: 3 g Protein: 30 g Calcium: 150 mg Fat: 22 g
Sugar: 2 g

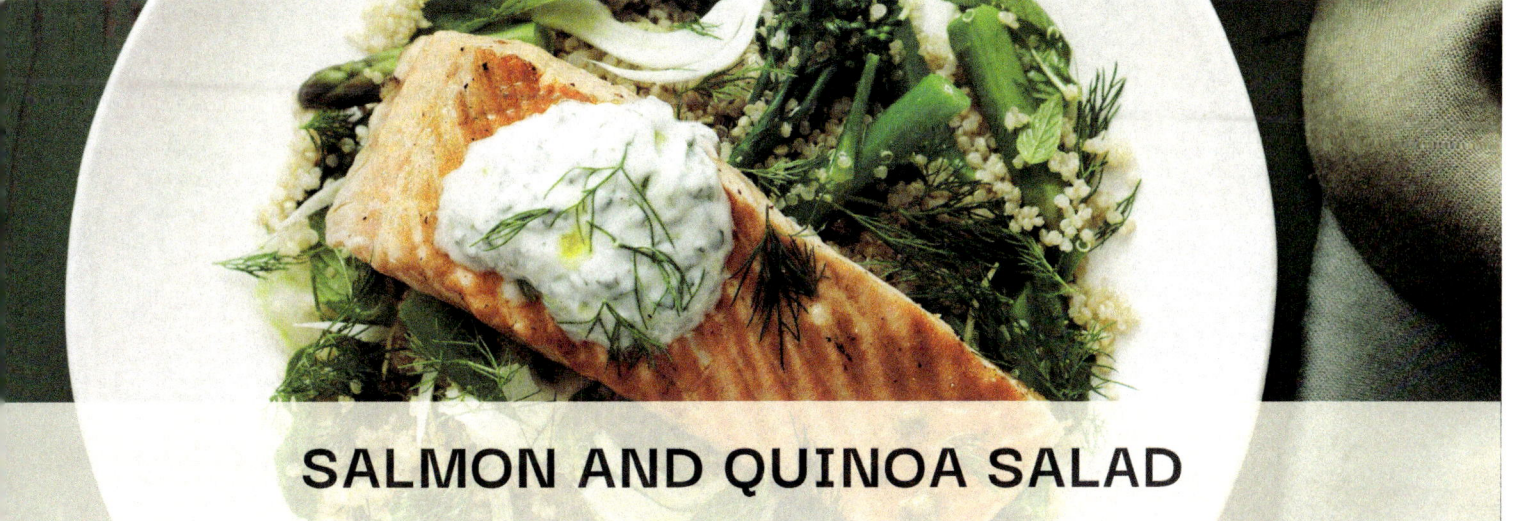

SALMON AND QUINOA SALAD

Salmon and Quinoa Salad is a wholesome and nutritious dish that combines protein-rich salmon with fluffy quinoa, fresh vegetables, and a zesty lemon dressing. It's perfect for a light lunch or a satisfying dinner, offering a balance of flavors and textures.

Serves	Preparation Time	Cooking Time
4	15 minutes	25 minute

Ingredients:

- 2 salmon fillets (about 6 oz each)
- 1 cup quinoa
- 2 cups water or vegetable broth
- 1 tablespoon olive oil
- Salt and black pepper to taste
- 1 cup cherry tomatoes, halved
- 1 cucumber, diced
- 1/4 red onion, thinly sliced
- 1/4 cup fresh parsley, chopped
- 2 tablespoons lemon juice
- 1 tablespoon olive oil (for dressing)
- 1 teaspoon Dijon mustard
- 1 teaspoon honey (optional)

Instructions:

1. **Cook the Quinoa:** Rinse the quinoa under cold water. In a medium saucepan, combine the quinoa and water (or broth) and bring to a boil. Reduce the heat to low, cover, and simmer for 15 minutes, or until the quinoa is cooked and the water is absorbed. Fluff the quinoa with a fork and let it cool slightly.
2. **Prepare the Salmon:** Preheat the oven to 375°F (190°C). Place the salmon fillets on a baking sheet lined with parchment paper. Drizzle with olive oil and season with salt and black pepper. Bake the salmon for 12-15 minutes, or until it flakes easily with a fork. Remove from the oven and let it cool slightly before flaking it into bite-sized pieces.
3. **Assemble the Salad:** In a large salad bowl, combine the cooked quinoa, cherry tomatoes, cucumber, red onion, and fresh parsley. Add the flaked salmon to the bowl.
4. **Prepare the Dressing:** In a small bowl, whisk together the lemon juice, olive oil, Dijon mustard, and honey (if using). Drizzle the dressing over the salad and toss gently to combine all the ingredients.
5. **Serve:** Divide the salad into serving bowls. Garnish with additional parsley or a lemon wedge if desired. Serve immediately, or refrigerate for up to 1 day for a chilled salad.

Nutrients (per serving)

Calories: 400 Sodium: 300 mg Carbohydrates: 28 g
Fiber: 5 g Protein: 30 g Calcium: 40 mg Fat: 18 g
Sugar: 4 g

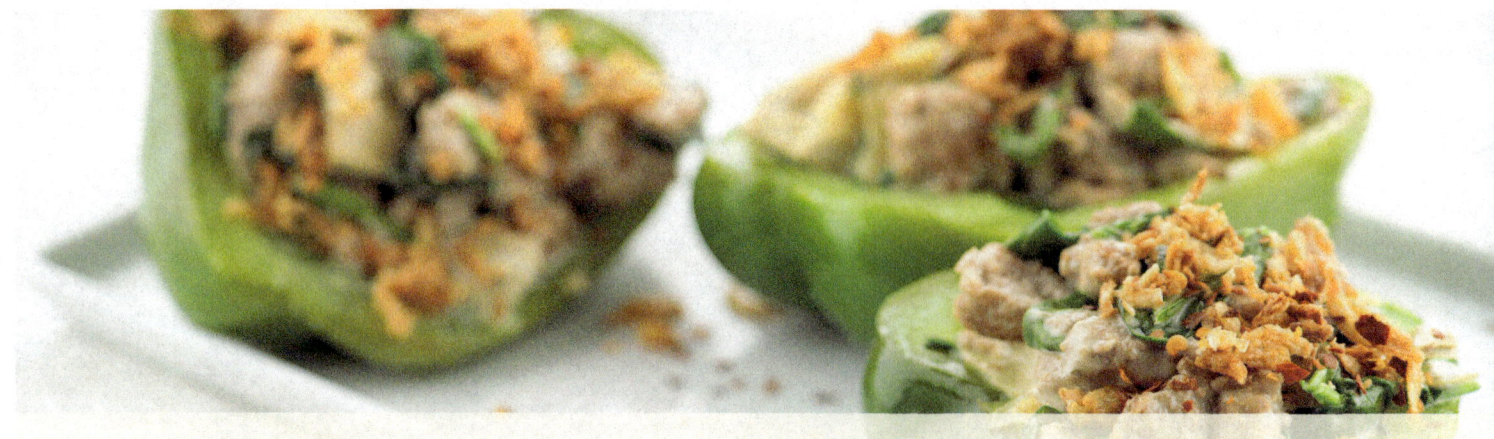

TURKEY AND SPINACH STUFFED PEPPERS

Turkey and Spinach Stuffed Peppers are a healthy and flavorful dish that combines lean ground turkey with nutrient-rich spinach, all baked inside sweet bell peppers. This recipe is perfect for a satisfying dinner that's both low in carbs and high in protein.

Serves	Preparation Time	Cooking Time 
4	15 minutes	35 minute

Ingredients:

- 4 large bell peppers (any color)
- 1 lb (450g) ground turkey
- 1 tablespoon olive oil
- 1 small onion, finely chopped
- 2 cloves garlic, minced
- 2 cups fresh spinach, chopped
- 1/2 cup cooked quinoa or brown rice (optional)
- 1 teaspoon dried oregano
- 1 teaspoon dried basil
- Salt and black pepper to taste
- 1/2 cup shredded mozzarella cheese (optional)

Instructions:

1. **Prepare the Peppers:** Preheat the oven to 375°F (190°C). Cut the tops off the bell peppers and remove the seeds and membranes. Lightly oil a baking dish and place the peppers upright in the dish. Set aside.
2. **Cook the Filling:** In a large skillet, heat the olive oil over medium heat. Add the chopped onion and garlic, sautéing until softened, about 3-4 minutes. Add the ground turkey to the skillet, breaking it apart with a spatula. Cook until browned and cooked through, about 7-8 minutes. Stir in the chopped spinach and cook until wilted, about 2 minutes. If using, stir in the cooked quinoa or brown rice. Season the mixture with oregano, basil, salt, and black pepper to taste. Remove from heat.
3. **Stuff the Peppers:** Spoon the turkey and spinach mixture into the prepared bell peppers, packing it down slightly. If desired, sprinkle the tops with shredded mozzarella cheese.
4. **Bake the Peppers:** Cover the baking dish with aluminum foil and bake in the preheated oven for 25 minutes. Remove the foil and bake for an additional 10 minutes, or until the peppers are tender and the cheese is melted and bubbly.
5. **Serve:** Let the stuffed peppers cool for a few minutes before serving. Serve with a side salad or steamed vegetables for a complete meal.

Nutrients (per serving)

Calories: 280   Sodium: 450 mg   Carbohydrates: 12 g
Fiber: 4 g   Protein: 28 g   Calcium: 80 mg   Fat: 12 g
Sugar: 5 g

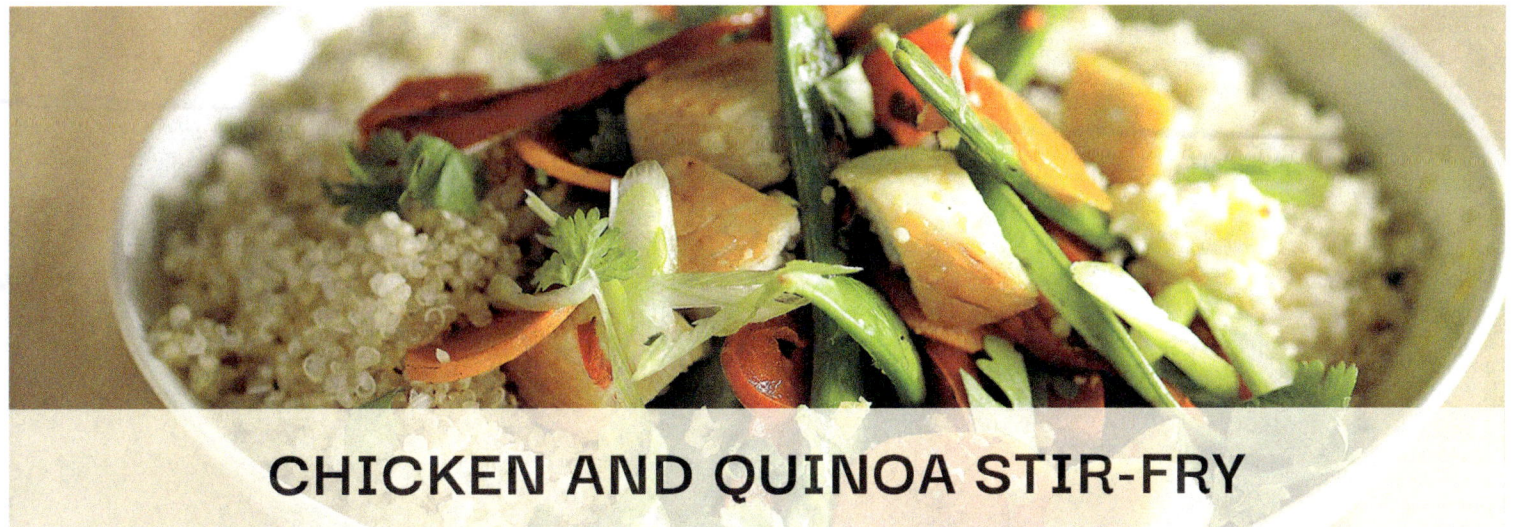

CHICKEN AND QUINOA STIR-FRY

Chicken and Quinoa Stir-Fry is a nutritious and quick meal, combining lean chicken breast with protein-packed quinoa and a variety of colorful vegetables. This dish is a great option for a balanced dinner that's both flavorful and satisfying.

Serves	Preparation Time	Cooking Time 
4	15 minutes	20 minute

Ingredients:

- 1 cup quinoa, uncooked
- 2 cups water or chicken broth
- 1 lb (450g) chicken breast, cut into bite-sized pieces
- 2 tablespoons olive oil
- 1 small onion, diced
- 2 cloves garlic, minced
- 1 red bell pepper, sliced
- 1 yellow bell pepper, sliced
- 1 medium zucchini, sliced
- 1 cup broccoli florets
- 2 tablespoons soy sauce (low-sodium)
- 1 tablespoon sesame oil
- 1 tablespoon grated ginger
- 1 tablespoon lime juice
- Salt and black pepper to taste
- Chopped green onions and sesame seeds for garnish (optional)

Instructions:

1. **Cook the Quinoa:** Rinse the quinoa under cold water. In a medium saucepan, combine quinoa and water or chicken broth. Bring to a boil, then reduce heat to low, cover, and simmer for 15 minutes, or until the quinoa is tender and water is absorbed. Fluff with a fork and set aside.
2. **Cook the Chicken:** In a large skillet or wok, heat 1 tablespoon of olive oil over medium-high heat. Add the chicken pieces and season with salt and black pepper. Cook for about 5-7 minutes, or until the chicken is browned and cooked through. Remove the chicken from the skillet and set aside.
3. **Sauté the Vegetables:** In the same skillet, add the remaining tablespoon of olive oil. Add the diced onion and minced garlic, sautéing until fragrant, about 2 minutes. Add the bell peppers, zucchini, and broccoli florets. Stir-fry the vegetables for 5-7 minutes, or until they are tender but still crisp.
4. **Combine and Stir-Fry:** Return the cooked chicken to the skillet with the vegetables. Add the cooked quinoa, soy sauce, sesame oil, grated ginger, and lime juice. Stir everything together and cook for another 2-3 minutes, allowing the flavors to meld. Adjust seasoning with additional salt and pepper if needed.
5. **Serve:** Transfer the stir-fry to a serving dish. Garnish with chopped green onions and sesame seeds, if desired. Serve hot and enjoy!

Nutrients (per serving)

Calories: 360 Sodium: 460 mg Carbohydrates: 30 g
Fiber: 5 g Protein: 30 g Calcium: 60 mg Fat: 14 g
Sugar: 4 g

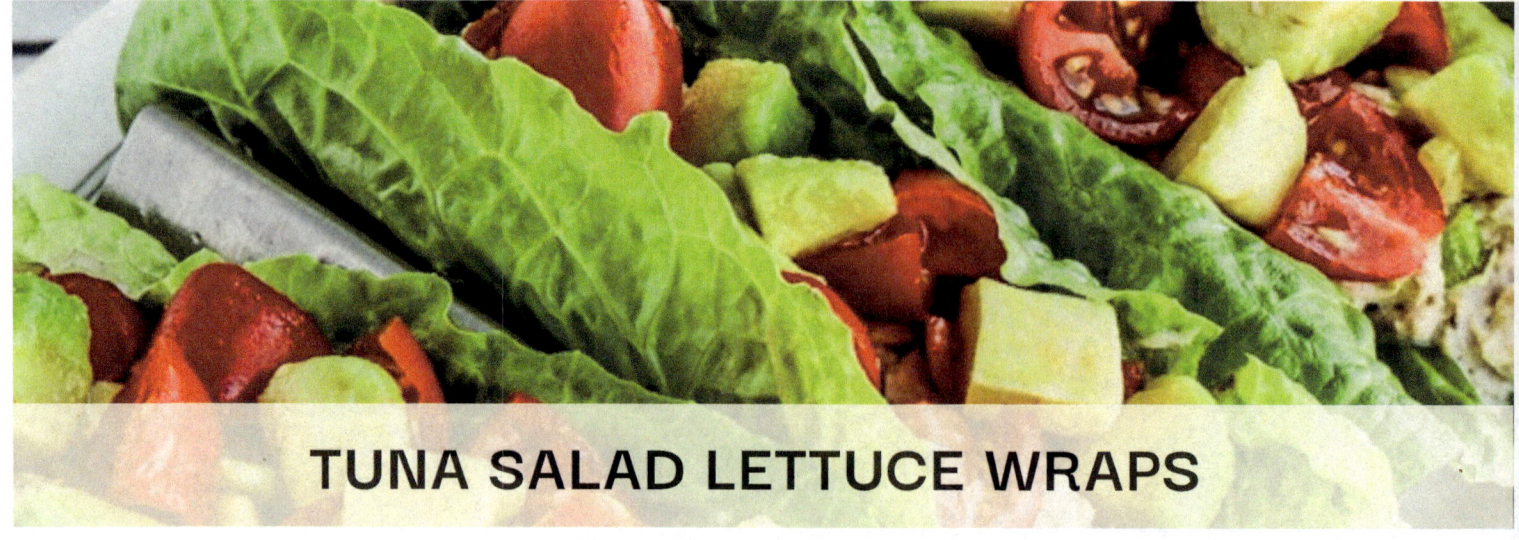

TUNA SALAD LETTUCE WRAPS

Tuna Salad Lettuce Wraps offer a refreshing and light alternative to traditional sandwiches. These wraps feature a flavorful tuna salad made with simple, wholesome ingredients, wrapped in crisp lettuce leaves for a low-carb, protein-packed meal.

Serves	Preparation Time	Cooking Time 
4	10 minutes	0 minute

Ingredients:

1 can (5 oz) tuna, drained
1/4 cup mayonnaise (or Greek yogurt for a lighter option)
1 tablespoon Dijon mustard
1 tablespoon lemon juice
1 celery stalk, finely chopped
1/4 small red onion, finely chopped
1 tablespoon capers, chopped (optional)
1 tablespoon fresh dill, chopped (or 1 teaspoon dried dill)
Salt and black pepper to taste
8-10 large lettuce leaves (such as Romaine or Butter Lettuce)

Instructions:

1. **Prepare the Tuna Salad:** In a medium bowl, combine the drained tuna, mayonnaise (or Greek yogurt), Dijon mustard, and lemon juice. Mix well. Add the chopped celery, red onion, capers (if using), and fresh dill. Stir to combine. Season with salt and black pepper to taste. Adjust seasoning if needed.
2. **Assemble the Wraps:** Wash and pat dry the lettuce leaves. Arrange them on a serving platter. Spoon a generous amount of the tuna salad onto each lettuce leaf. Fold the sides of the lettuce over the filling to create a wrap.
3. **Serve:** Arrange the lettuce wraps on a serving platter. Serve immediately or refrigerate until ready to serve.

Nutrients (per serving)

Calories: 180 Sodium: 480 mg Carbohydrates: 5 g
Fiber: 2 g Protein: 22 g Calcium: 40 mg Fat: 10 g
Sugar: 1 g

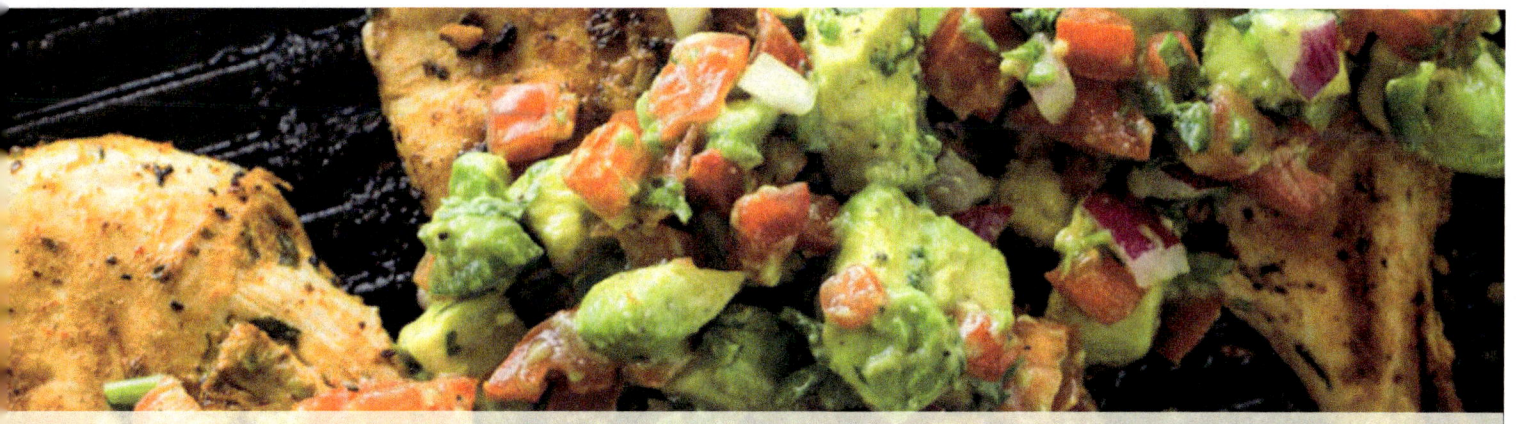

GRILLED CHICKEN WITH AVOCADO SALSA

Grilled Chicken with Avocado Salsa is a vibrant and flavorful dish that's perfect for a healthy meal. The grilled chicken is paired with a fresh avocado salsa that adds a creamy texture and a burst of flavor, making it a delicious and nutritious choice for any time of the day.

Serves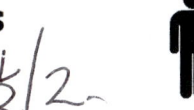
4 ~~5~~/2-

Preparation Time
15 minutes

Cooking Time
15 minute

Ingredients:

For the Chicken:
- 4 boneless, skinless chicken breasts
- 2 tablespoons olive oil
- 1 tablespoon smoked paprika
- 1 teaspoon garlic powder
- 1 teaspoon onion powder
- 1 teaspoon dried oregano
- Salt and black pepper to taste

For the Avocado Salsa:
- 2 ripe avocados, diced
- 1 cup cherry tomatoes, halved
- 1/4 red onion, finely chopped
- ~~1 jalapeño, seeded and minced (optional, for heat)~~
- 2 tablespoons fresh cilantro, chopped
- 1 tablespoon lime juice
- Salt and black pepper to taste

or griddle.

Instructions:

1. **Prepare the Chicken:** Preheat the grill to medium-high heat. In a small bowl, mix together olive oil, smoked paprika, garlic powder, onion powder, dried oregano, salt, and black pepper. Rub the spice mixture evenly over the chicken breasts. Grill the chicken for 6-7 minutes per side, or until the internal temperature reaches 165°F (74°C) and the chicken is cooked through. Remove from the grill and let rest for 5 minutes before slicing.
2. **Prepare the Avocado Salsa:** In a medium bowl, combine the diced avocados, cherry tomatoes, red onion, jalapeño (if using), cilantro, and lime juice. Gently toss to combine and season with salt and black pepper to taste.
3. **Serve:** Slice the grilled chicken breasts and arrange them on a serving platter. Top with the avocado salsa. Serve immediately.

Nutrients (per serving)

Calories: 320 Sodium: 150 mg Carbohydrates: 14 g

Fiber: 6 g Protein: 30 g Calcium: 40 mg Fat: 18 g

Sugar: 3 g

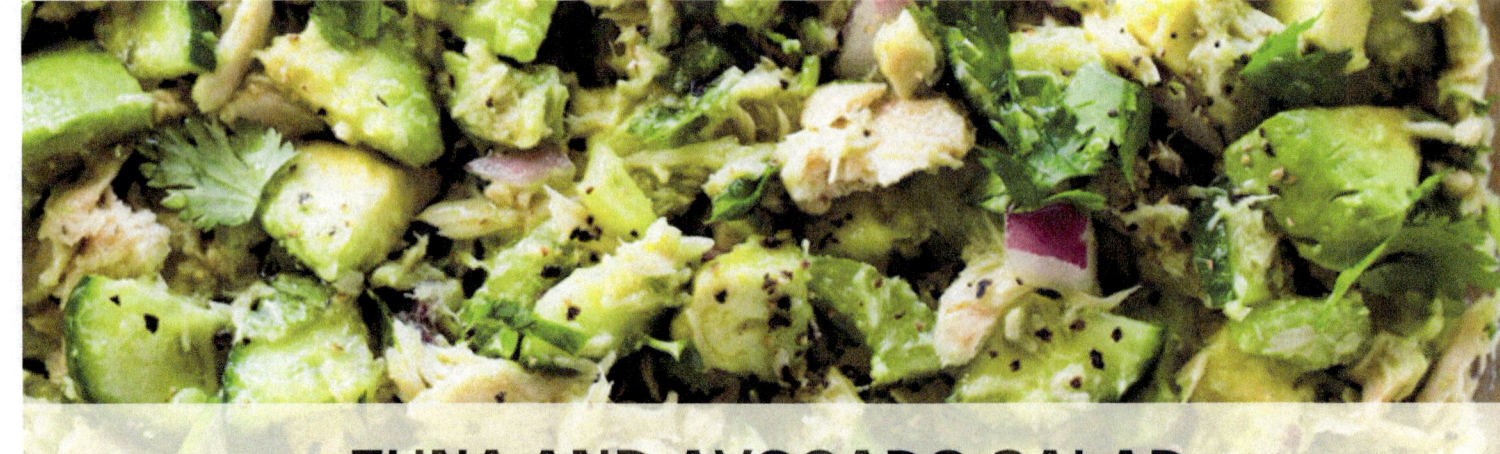

TUNA AND AVOCADO SALAD

Tuna and Avocado Salad is a refreshing and nutritious dish that's perfect for a quick lunch or a light dinner. Combining the creamy texture of avocado with the protein-packed tuna, this salad is both satisfying and full of flavor.

Serves	Preparation Time	Cooking Time
4 ½ /2. 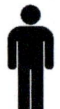	10 minutes	0 minute 

Ingredients:

- ✓ 1 can (5 oz) tuna, drained
- ½ 1 ripe avocado, diced
- ✓ 1/2 cup cherry tomatoes, halved
- ⅛ 1/4 cucumber, diced
- Slice 1/4 red onion, finely chopped
- 1 2 tablespoons fresh parsley or cilantro, chopped
- 1 2 tablespoons olive oil
- ½ 1 tablespoon lemon juice
- Salt and black pepper to taste

Instructions:

1. **Prepare the Salad:** In a large bowl, combine the drained tuna, diced avocado, cherry tomatoes, cucumber, red onion, and chopped parsley or cilantro.
2. **Make the Dressing:** In a small bowl, whisk together olive oil, lemon juice, salt, and black pepper.
3. **Assemble the Salad:** Drizzle the dressing over the tuna and avocado mixture. Gently toss to combine, ensuring the salad ingredients are evenly coated with the dressing.
4. **Serve:** Serve immediately or refrigerate until ready to serve.

on leaves.
New potatoes.

Nutrients (per serving)

Calories: 250 Sodium: 300 mg Carbohydrates: 12 g
Fiber: 6 g Protein: 18 g Calcium: 40 mg Fat: 15 g
Sugar: 2 g

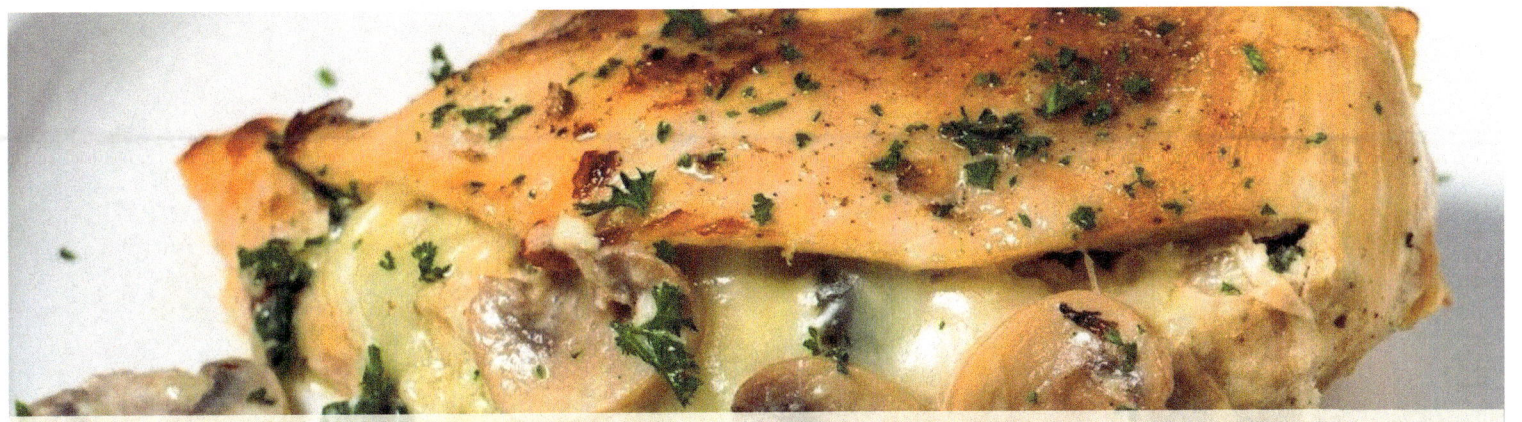

CHICKEN AND SPINACH STUFFED MUSHROOMS

Chicken and Spinach Stuffed Mushrooms are a flavorful and nutritious dish that makes for a great appetizer or a light main course. These mushrooms are filled with a savory mixture of chicken and spinach, creating a delightful combination of textures and tastes.

Serves 	Preparation Time	Cooking Time 
4	15 minutes	20 minute

Ingredients:

12 large white or cremini mushrooms, stems removed and cleaned
1 cup cooked chicken, finely chopped (about 1-2 chicken breasts)
1 cup fresh spinach, chopped
1/4 cup grated Parmesan cheese
1/4 cup cream cheese, softened
1/4 cup breadcrumbs (optional, for added texture)
2 cloves garlic, minced
1 tablespoon olive oil
1/4 teaspoon dried oregano
Salt and black pepper to taste
Fresh parsley, chopped (for garnish)

Instructions:

1. **Prepare the Filling:** Preheat the oven to 375°F (190°C). Heat olive oil in a skillet over medium heat. Add minced garlic and cook for 1-2 minutes until fragrant. Add the chopped spinach and cook until wilted, about 2-3 minutes. Remove from heat. In a bowl, combine the cooked chicken, sautéed spinach, Parmesan cheese, cream cheese, breadcrumbs (if using), dried oregano, salt, and black pepper. Mix until well combined.
2. **Stuff the Mushrooms:** Arrange the mushroom caps on a baking sheet lined with parchment paper. Spoon the chicken and spinach mixture into each mushroom cap, pressing it down gently to pack the filling.
3. **Bake:** Bake in the preheated oven for 15-20 minutes, or until the mushrooms are tender and the filling is golden brown on top.
4. **Serve:** Garnish with freshly chopped parsley before serving. Serve warm as an appetizer or light meal.

Nutrients (per serving)

Calories: 190 Sodium: 350 mg Carbohydrates: 10 g
Fiber: 2 g Protein: 16 g Calcium: 140 mg Fat: 12 g
Sugar: 2 g

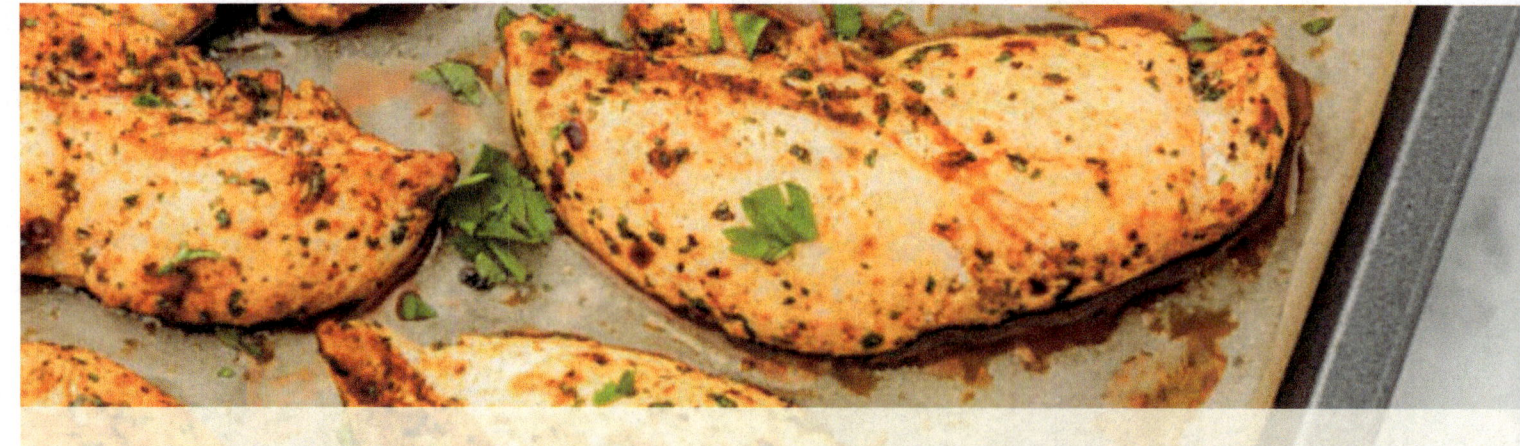

OVEN-BAKED CHICKEN TENDERS

Oven-Baked Chicken Tenders are a healthier alternative to fried chicken tenders. Crispy on the outside and tender on the inside, these chicken tenders are coated in a flavorful breadcrumb mixture and baked to perfection. They make a great snack, appetizer, or main dish for the whole family.

Serves 	Preparation Time	Cooking Time 
4	15 minutes	20 minute

Ingredients:

1 lb (450 g) chicken tenders (or chicken breast cut into strips)
1 cup whole wheat breadcrumbs (or panko breadcrumbs for extra crunch)
1/2 cup grated Parmesan cheese
1 teaspoon paprika
1/2 teaspoon garlic powder
1/2 teaspoon onion powder
1/2 teaspoon dried oregano
1/2 teaspoon dried thyme
Salt and black pepper to taste
1/4 cup all-purpose flour G/F.
2 large eggs
Cooking spray or olive oil for spraying

Instructions:

1. **Prepare the Breading:** Preheat the oven to 400°F (200°C). Line a baking sheet with parchment paper or lightly grease it with cooking spray.In a shallow bowl, mix together the breadcrumbs, Parmesan cheese, paprika, garlic powder, onion powder, dried oregano, dried thyme, salt, and black pepper.Place the flour in a separate shallow bowl.In another bowl, beat the eggs.
2. **Bread the Chicken:** Dredge each chicken tender in the flour, shaking off any excess.Dip the floured chicken into the beaten eggs, allowing any excess to drip off.Coat the chicken with the breadcrumb mixture, pressing gently to adhere the crumbs.
3. **Bake the Tenders:** Arrange the breaded chicken tenders on the prepared baking sheet in a single layer.Lightly spray or brush the tops of the tenders with cooking spray or olive oil.Bake in the preheated oven for 15-20 minutes, or until the tenders are golden brown and cooked through (internal temperature should reach 165°F or 74°C).
4. **Serve:** Serve the chicken tenders warm with your favorite dipping sauces or a side of vegetables.

Nutrients (per serving)

Calories: 280 Sodium: 500 mg Carbohydrates: 15 g
Fiber: 2 g Protein: 25 g Calcium: 150 mg Fat: 12 g
Sugar: 1 g

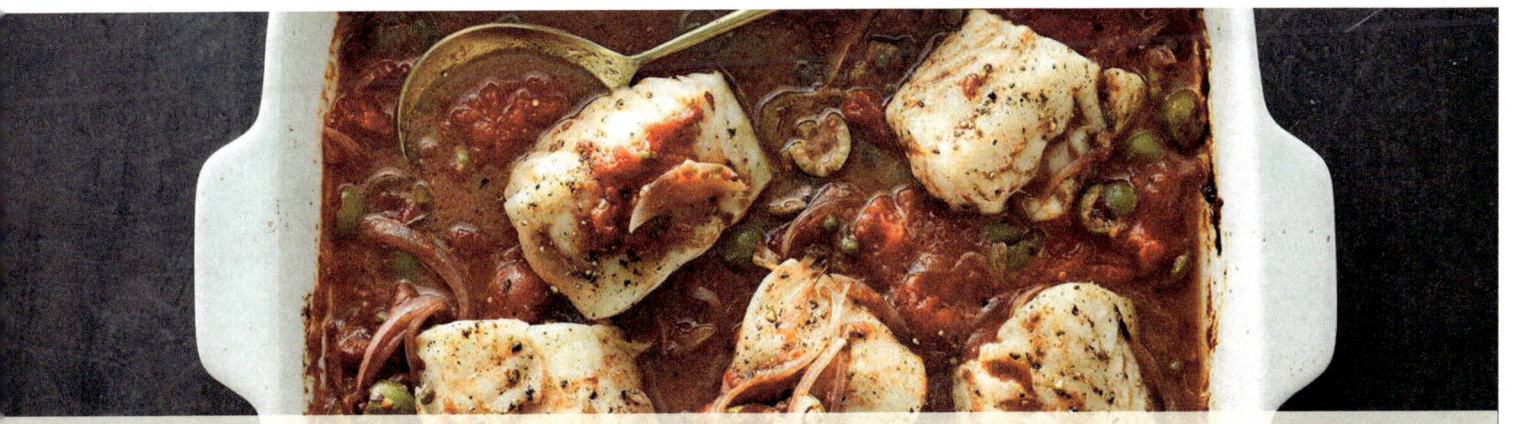

BAKED COD WITH TOMATOES AND OLIVES

Baked Cod with Tomatoes and Olives is a simple yet flavorful dish that combines tender cod fillets with a savory mix of tomatoes, olives, and herbs. This Mediterranean-inspired recipe is perfect for a healthy weeknight dinner, offering a balance of fresh flavors and nutritious ingredients.

Serves
4 1/2/2.

Preparation Time
10 minutes

Cooking Time
20 minute

Ingredients:

4 cod fillets (about 6 oz each) 2 100-120g
1 cup cherry tomatoes, halved   1/4
1/2 cup black olives, pitted and sliced
2 cloves garlic, minced   1
1 tablespoon olive oil   1/2
1 teaspoon dried oregano   1/2 1/2
1 teaspoon dried basil   1/2
1/2 teaspoon dried thyme   1/4
Salt and black pepper to taste
Fresh parsley, chopped (for garnish)
Lemon wedges (for serving)

Instructions:

1. **Prepare the Oven:** Preheat the oven to 400°F (200°C). Lightly grease a baking dish or line it with parchment paper.
2. **Prepare the Vegetables:** In a bowl, toss the cherry tomatoes, sliced olives, minced garlic, olive oil, dried oregano, dried basil, dried thyme, salt, and black pepper.
3. **Assemble the Dish:** Arrange the cod fillets in a single layer in the prepared baking dish. Spoon the tomato and olive mixture over the cod fillets, spreading it evenly.
4. **Bake:** Bake in the preheated oven for 15-20 minutes, or until the cod is cooked through and flakes easily with a fork. The internal temperature should reach 145°F (63°C).
5. **Serve:** Garnish with freshly chopped parsley. Serve with lemon wedges on the side for a burst of fresh flavor.

Preheat A/F 180.
15-20m.

Nutrients (per serving)

Calories: 220 Sodium: 300 mg Carbohydrates: 10 g
Fiber: 2 g Protein: 30 g Calcium: 60 mg Fat: 8 g
Sugar: 5 g

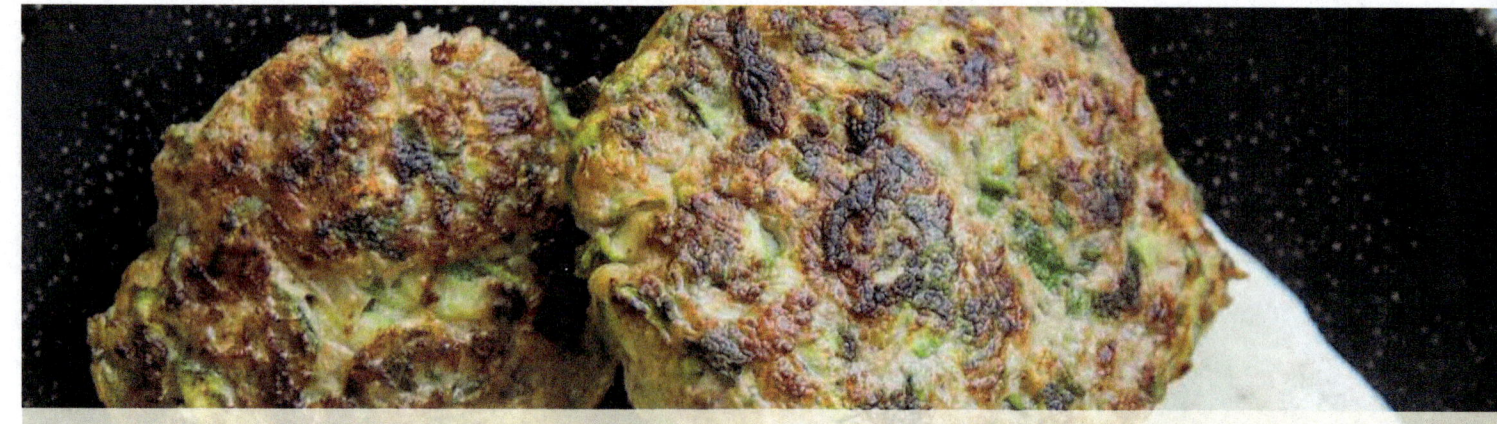

TURKEY AND ~~ZUCCHINI~~ BURGERS
chicken

Turkey and Zucchini Burgers are a light and nutritious alternative to traditional beef burgers. The addition of grated zucchini keeps these burgers moist and adds extra vegetables to your meal. They're perfect for a healthy weeknight dinner or a casual outdoor BBQ.

Frozen Chicken mince - Big Iceland.

Serves	Preparation Time	Cooking Time
4	15 minutes	12 minute

Ingredients:

- 1 lb (450 g) ground ~~turkey~~ *chicken*
- 1 cup grated zucchini (excess moisture squeezed out) *(1 courgette)*
- 1/4 cup finely chopped onion *small onion*
- 2 cloves garlic, minced
- ✓ 1/4 cup whole wheat breadcrumbs *GF or panko.*
- ✓ 1 large egg
- ✓ 1 tablespoon chopped fresh parsley
- ✓ 1 teaspoon dried oregano
- ✓ 1/2 teaspoon ground cumin
- ✓ Salt and black pepper to taste
- Cooking spray or olive oil for grilling

Instructions:

1. **Prepare the Mixture:** In a large bowl, combine the ground turkey, grated zucchini, chopped onion, minced garlic, breadcrumbs, egg, parsley, oregano, cumin, salt, and black pepper. Mix until all ingredients are well incorporated.
2. **Form the Patties:** Divide the mixture into 4 equal portions and shape them into patties, about 1/2 inch thick.
3. **Cook the Burgers:** Heat a grill or skillet over medium heat and lightly coat with cooking spray or olive oil. Cook the patties for about 5-6 minutes on each side, or until the internal temperature reaches 165°F (74°C) and the burgers are cooked through. → *8 mins each side*
4. **Serve:** Serve the burgers warm on whole wheat buns or lettuce wraps, with your favorite toppings and condiments.

Use burger press.

Tasty!

Make 6 next time.

*cook **all***

mustn't re-freeze mince without cooking, then re-heat/ AIF.

220 × 4 = 880 ÷ 6 = 146c.

Nutrients (per serving)

Calories: 220 Sodium: 250 mg Carbohydrates: 10 g
Fiber: 2 g Protein: 28 g Calcium: 30 mg Fat: 8 g
Sugar: 2 g

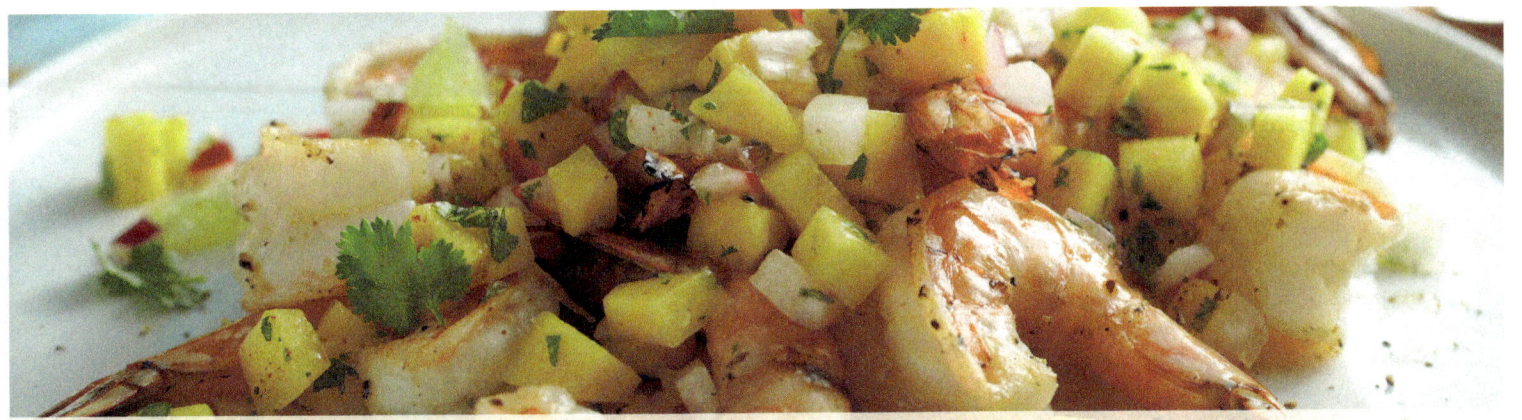

GRILLED SHRIMP WITH MANGO SALSA

Grilled Shrimp with Mango Salsa is a vibrant and refreshing dish that combines smoky grilled shrimp with a sweet and tangy mango salsa. Perfect for a light dinner or a summer BBQ, this dish is both flavorful and easy to prepare, bringing a taste of the tropics to your table.

Serves	Preparation Time	Cooking Time 
4	20 minutes	6 minute

Ingredients:

For the Shrimp:

1 lb (450 g) large shrimp, peeled and deveined
2 tablespoons olive oil
1 tablespoon lime juice
2 cloves garlic, minced
1 teaspoon paprika
1/2 teaspoon ground cumin
Salt and black pepper to taste

For the Mango Salsa:

1 ripe mango, peeled, pitted, and diced
1/2 red bell pepper, finely chopped
1/4 cup red onion, finely chopped
1 jalapeño, seeded and minced (optional for heat)
2 tablespoons fresh cilantro, chopped
1 tablespoon lime juice
Salt to taste

Instructions:

1. **Marinate the Shrimp:** In a bowl, combine the olive oil, lime juice, minced garlic, paprika, ground cumin, salt, and black pepper. Add the shrimp and toss to coat evenly. Marinate for at least 15 minutes.
2. **Prepare the Mango Salsa:** In a medium bowl, mix together the diced mango, red bell pepper, red onion, jalapeño (if using), cilantro, lime juice, and a pinch of salt. Stir gently to combine and set aside.
3. **Grill the Shrimp:** Preheat the grill to medium-high heat. If using skewers, thread the shrimp onto them. Grill the shrimp for 2-3 minutes on each side, or until they turn pink and are cooked through. Be careful not to overcook.
4. **Serve:** Arrange the grilled shrimp on a serving platter and top with mango salsa. Serve immediately, garnished with additional cilantro if desired.

Nutrients (per serving)

Calories: 220 Sodium: 300 mg Carbohydrates: 15 g
Fiber: 2 g Protein: 20 g Calcium: 50 mg Fat: 10 g
Sugar: 12 g

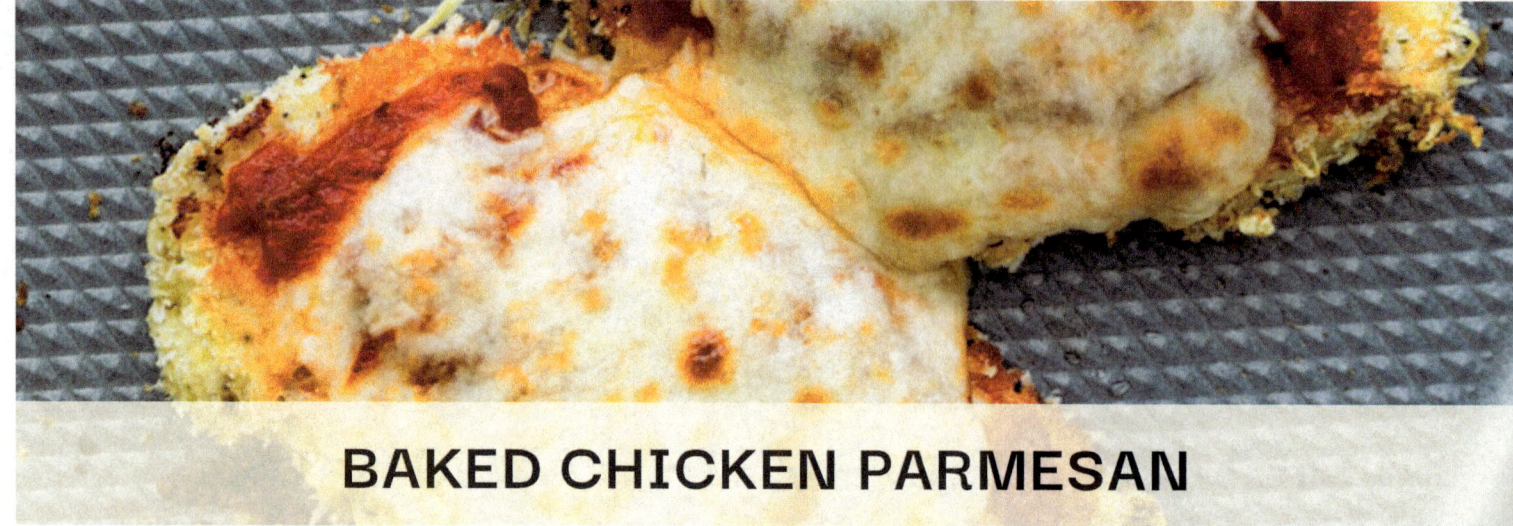

BAKED CHICKEN PARMESAN

Baked Chicken Parmesan is a healthier twist on the classic Italian favorite. This dish features breaded and baked chicken breasts topped with marinara sauce and melted cheese, providing all the delicious flavors of traditional Chicken Parmesan with less fat and fewer calories.

Serves	Preparation Time	Cooking Time
4	15 minutes	25 minute

Ingredients:

4 boneless, skinless chicken breasts (about 6 oz each)
1 cup whole wheat breadcrumbs
1/2 cup grated Parmesan cheese
1 teaspoon dried basil
1 teaspoon dried oregano
1/2 teaspoon garlic powder
1/2 teaspoon onion powder
Salt and black pepper to taste
1 large egg
1 cup marinara sauce (preferably low-sugar)
1 cup shredded mozzarella cheese
Fresh basil leaves (for garnish)

Instructions:

1. **Prepare the Oven:** Preheat the oven to 400°F (200°C). Lightly grease a baking sheet or line it with parchment paper.
2. **Prepare the Coating:** In a shallow dish, combine the whole wheat breadcrumbs, grated Parmesan cheese, dried basil, dried oregano, garlic powder, onion powder, salt, and black pepper. In another shallow dish, beat the egg.
3. **Coat the Chicken:** Dip each chicken breast into the beaten egg, allowing any excess to drip off. Coat the chicken breast with the breadcrumb mixture, pressing lightly to adhere. Place the coated chicken breasts on the prepared baking sheet.
4. **Bake the Chicken:** Bake in the preheated oven for 20-25 minutes, or until the chicken reaches an internal temperature of 165°F (74°C) and the coating is golden brown and crispy.
5. **Add Sauce and Cheese:** Remove the baking sheet from the oven. Spoon about 2 tablespoons of marinara sauce over each chicken breast. Sprinkle shredded mozzarella cheese on top of the sauce.
6. **Broil for Finish:** Return the baking sheet to the oven and broil on high for 2-3 minutes, or until the cheese is melted and bubbly. Watch carefully to avoid burning.
7. **Serve:** Garnish with fresh basil leaves and serve immediately.

Nutrients (per serving)

Calories: 350 Sodium: 700 mg Carbohydrates: 20 g
Fiber: 3 g Protein: 40 g Calcium: 300 mg Fat: 14 g
Sugar: 6 g

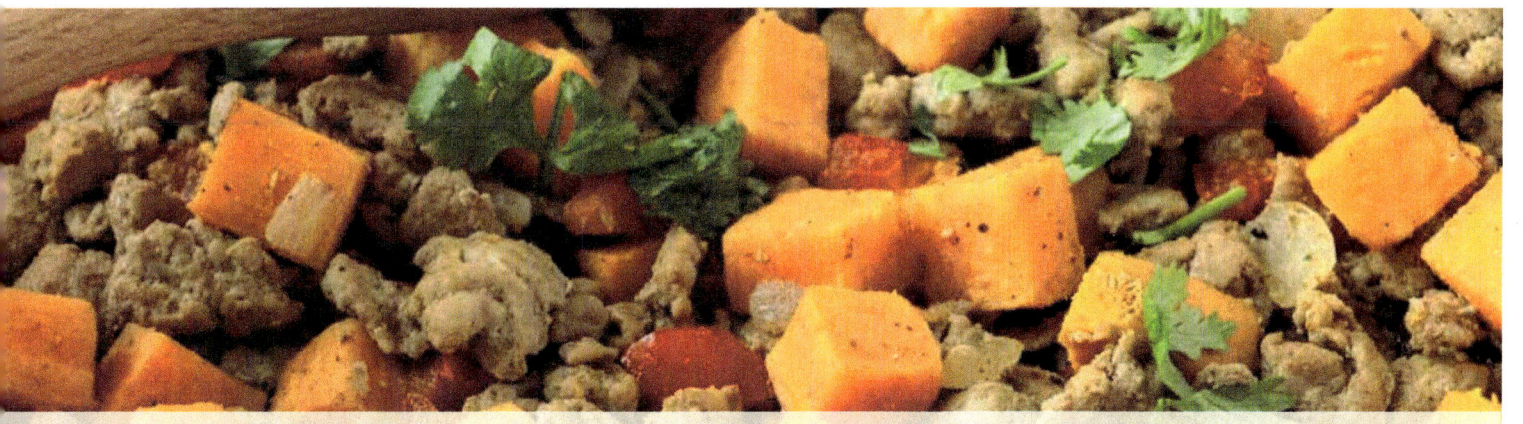

TURKEY AND SWEET POTATO HASH

Turkey and Sweet Potato Hash is a hearty and nutritious dish that's perfect for a satisfying breakfast or a light dinner. Combining lean ground turkey with sweet potatoes and a blend of vegetables, this hash is full of flavor and packed with nutrients.

Serves	Preparation Time	Cooking Time 
4	15 minutes	20 minute

Ingredients:

1 lb (450 g) ground ~~turkey~~ Chicken
2 medium sweet potatoes, peeled and diced
1 red bell pepper, diced
1 onion, diced
2 cloves garlic, minced
1 teaspoon paprika
1/2 teaspoon ground cumin
1/2 teaspoon dried thyme
Salt and black pepper to taste
2 tablespoons olive oil
2 tablespoons fresh parsley, chopped (for garnish)

Instructions:

1. **Cook the Sweet Potatoes:** Heat 1 tablespoon of olive oil in a large skillet over medium heat. Add the diced sweet potatoes and cook, stirring occasionally, for about 10-12 minutes, or until they are tender and lightly browned. Remove from the skillet and set aside.
2. **Cook the Turkey:** In the same skillet, add the remaining tablespoon of olive oil. Add the diced onion and cook until it becomes translucent, about 3-4 minutes. Stir in the minced garlic and cook for an additional 1 minute.
3. **Add the Turkey:** Add the ground turkey to the skillet. Cook, breaking it up with a spoon, until it is fully cooked and browned, about 6-8 minutes.
4. **Season and Combine:** Stir in the paprika, ground cumin, dried thyme, salt, and black pepper. Add the cooked sweet potatoes and diced red bell pepper to the skillet. Stir to combine and cook for an additional 3-4 minutes, or until everything is heated through and the flavors are well mixed.
5. **Serve:** Garnish with fresh parsley and serve warm.

Nutrients (per serving)

Calories: 350 Sodium: 250 mg Carbohydrates: 30 g
Fiber: 5 g Protein: 25 g Calcium: 70 mg Fat: 15 g
Sugar: 7 g

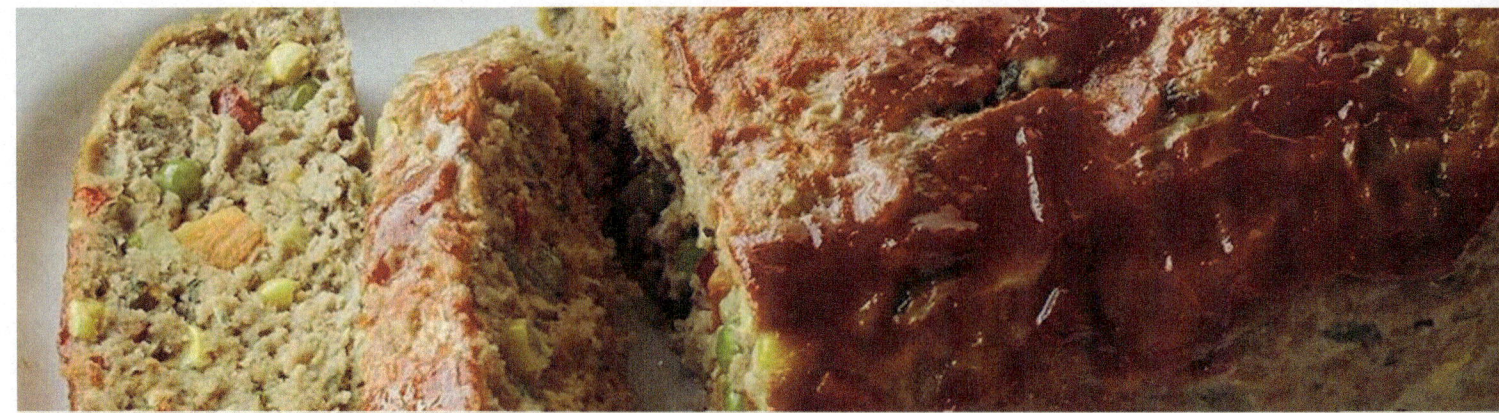

TURKEY AND VEGETABLE MEATLOAF

Turkey and Vegetable Meatloaf is a wholesome and flavorful dish that offers a lighter alternative to traditional meatloaf. Packed with lean ground turkey and a variety of vegetables, it's perfect for a nutritious family meal.

Serves  **Preparation Time** **Cooking Time**
4 15 minutes 60 minute

Ingredients:

1 lb (450 g) ground ~~turkey~~ *mince chicken.*
1 cup grated zucchini (water squeezed out)
1 cup finely chopped mushrooms
1/2 cup finely chopped onion
1/2 cup grated carrots
2 cloves garlic, minced
1 large egg
1/2 cup whole wheat breadcrumbs — *G/F / panko.*
1/4 cup grated ~~Parmesan~~ cheese *gran padano*
2 tablespoons tomato paste
1 tablespoon Worcestershire sauce
1 teaspoon dried thyme
1/2 teaspoon dried oregano
Salt and black pepper to taste
~~1/2 cup ketchup (for topping)~~

Instructions:

1. **Preheat Oven:** Preheat the oven to 375°F (190°C). Lightly grease a loaf pan or line it with parchment paper.
2. **Prepare Vegetables:** In a large mixing bowl, combine the grated zucchini, finely chopped mushrooms, chopped onion, grated carrots, and minced garlic.
3. **Mix Ingredients:** Add the ground turkey, egg, whole wheat breadcrumbs, grated Parmesan cheese, tomato paste, Worcestershire sauce, dried thyme, dried oregano, salt, and black pepper to the bowl. Mix until well combined.
4. **Form the Meatloaf:** Transfer the mixture to the prepared loaf pan and press it down evenly.
5. **Add Topping:** ~~Spread the ketchup evenly over the top of the meatloaf.~~
6. **Bake:** Bake in the preheated oven for 50-60 minutes, or until the meatloaf reaches an internal temperature of 165°F (74°C) and is cooked through.
7. **Cool and Serve:** Let the meatloaf cool in the pan for 10 minutes before slicing. Serve warm.

Nutrients (per serving)

Calories: 250 Sodium: 400 mg Carbohydrates: 20 g
Fiber: 3 g Protein: 25 g Calcium: 120 mg Fat: 10 g
Sugar: 6 g

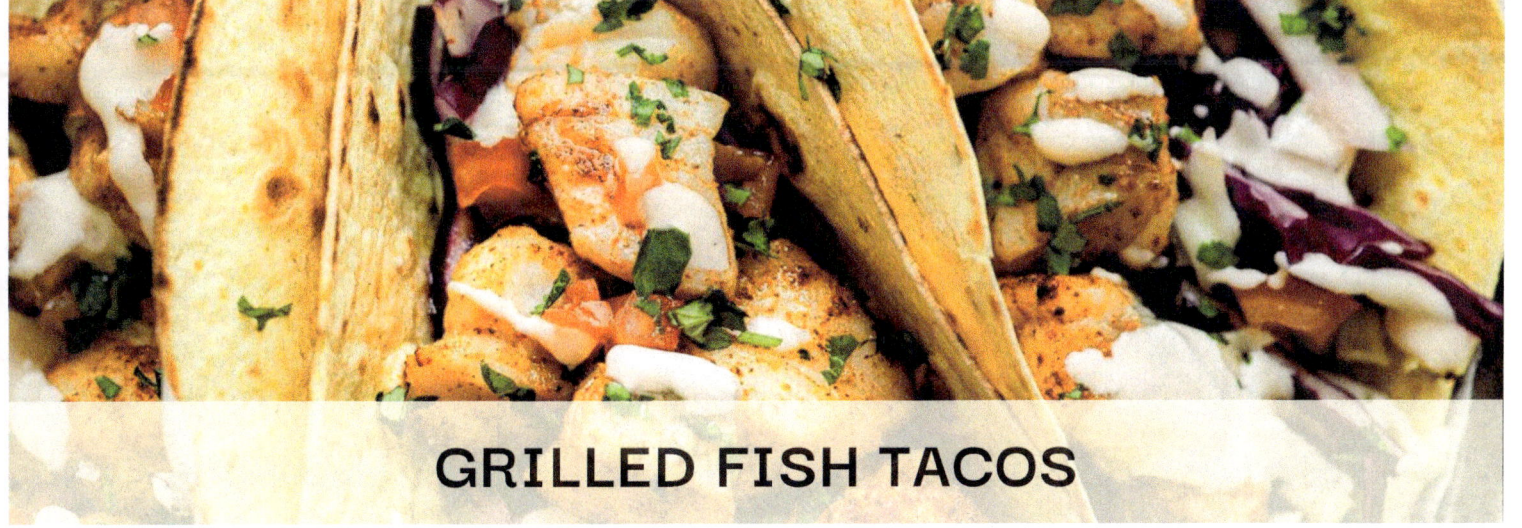

GRILLED FISH TACOS

Grilled Fish Tacos are a delicious and light meal that brings a taste of summer to your plate. Featuring tender, grilled fish and fresh toppings, these tacos are perfect for a quick weeknight dinner or a casual gathering.

Serves 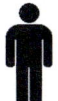	Preparation Time	Cooking Time 
4	15 minutes	10 minute

Ingredients:

1 lb (450 g) white fish fillets (such as tilapia, cod, or halibut)
2 tablespoons olive oil
1 tablespoon lime juice
1 teaspoon ground cumin
1 teaspoon smoked paprika
1/2 teaspoon garlic powder
1/2 teaspoon onion powder
Salt and black pepper to taste
8 small corn tortillas
1 cup shredded cabbage
1/2 cup diced tomatoes
1/4 cup chopped fresh cilantro
1/4 cup thinly sliced red onion
1 avocado, sliced
Lime wedges (for serving)

Instructions:

1. **Prepare the Fish:** In a small bowl, combine olive oil, lime juice, ground cumin, smoked paprika, garlic powder, onion powder, salt, and black pepper. Rub the spice mixture evenly over both sides of the fish fillets.
2. **Grill the Fish:** Preheat your grill to medium-high heat. Place the fish fillets on the grill and cook for 3-4 minutes per side, or until the fish is opaque and flakes easily with a fork. Remove from the grill and let rest for a few minutes.
3. **Prepare the Toppings:** While the fish is grilling, prepare the taco toppings: shred the cabbage, dice the tomatoes, chop the cilantro, and slice the red onion and avocado.
4. **Warm the Tortillas:** Heat the corn tortillas on the grill or in a dry skillet over medium heat until they are warm and pliable.
5. **Assemble the Tacos:** Flake the grilled fish into bite-sized pieces. Place a few pieces of fish on each tortilla. Top with shredded cabbage, diced tomatoes, chopped cilantro, sliced red onion, and avocado.
6. **Serve:** Serve the tacos with lime wedges on the side for squeezing over the top.

Nutrients (per serving)

Calories: 150 Sodium: 200 mg Carbohydrates: 15 g
Fiber: 4 g Protein: 12 g Calcium: 80 mg Fat: 7 g
Sugar: 2 g

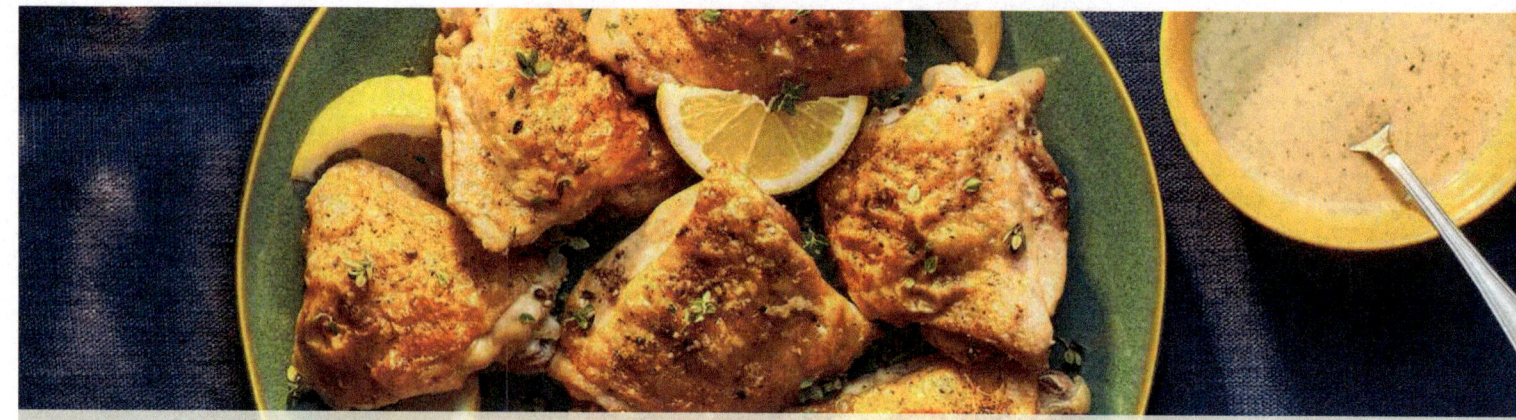

BAKED CHICKEN THIGHS WITH LEMON

Baked Chicken Thighs with Lemon is a simple yet flavorful dish that highlights the tangy brightness of lemon paired with tender, juicy chicken thighs. This easy recipe is perfect for a weeknight dinner or a satisfying meal prep option.

Serves 	Preparation Time	Cooking Time 
4	10 minutes	35 minute

Ingredients:

- 4 bone-in, skinless chicken thighs *2 cutlets / 2 breast*
- 2 tablespoons olive oil
- 2 tablespoons lemon juice
- 1 teaspoon lemon zest
- 4 cloves garlic, minced
- 1 teaspoon dried thyme
- 1 teaspoon dried rosemary
- 1 teaspoon paprika
- Salt and black pepper to taste
- Lemon slices (for garnish)
- Fresh parsley (for garnish, optional)

Instructions:

1. **Preheat Oven:** Preheat your oven to 400°F (200°C). Line a baking sheet with parchment paper or lightly grease it.
2. **Prepare the Marinade:** In a small bowl, whisk together olive oil, lemon juice, lemon zest, minced garlic, dried thyme, dried rosemary, paprika, salt, and black pepper.
3. **Marinate the Chicken:** Pat the chicken thighs dry with paper towels. Place them in a large bowl or resealable bag. Pour the marinade over the chicken and toss to coat evenly. Let the chicken marinate for at least 15 minutes or up to 2 hours in the refrigerator for best flavor.
4. **Bake the Chicken:** Arrange the marinated chicken thighs on the prepared baking sheet. Bake in the preheated oven for 30-35 minutes, or until the chicken reaches an internal temperature of 165°F (74°C) and the skin is golden brown and crispy.
5. **Serve:** Garnish the baked chicken thighs with lemon slices and fresh parsley, if desired. Serve warm.

Nutrients (per serving)

Calories: 280 Sodium: 150 mg Carbohydrates: 2 g

Fiber: 1 g Protein: 24 g Calcium: 20 mg Fat: 20 g

Sugar: 1 g

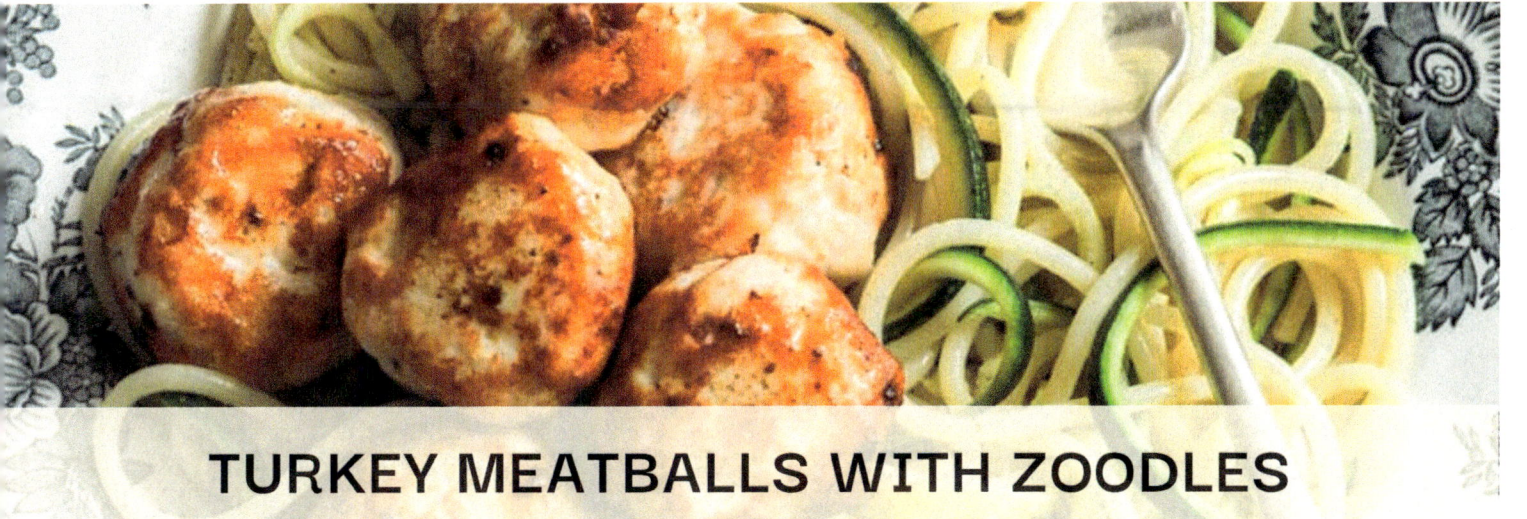

TURKEY MEATBALLS WITH ZOODLES

Turkey Meatballs with Zoodles is a healthy, low-carb meal that combines juicy turkey meatballs with fresh zucchini noodles. This dish is flavorful and satisfying, perfect for a nutritious weeknight dinner or meal prep.

Serves 	Preparation Time	Cooking Time 
4	15 minutes	25 minute

Ingredients:

For the Turkey Meatballs:
- 1 lb (450 g) ground turkey
- 1/4 cup grated Parmesan cheese
- 1/4 cup finely chopped parsley
- 1/4 cup finely chopped onion
- 1 egg
- 2 cloves garlic, minced
- 1/2 teaspoon dried oregano
- 1/2 teaspoon dried basil
- Salt and black pepper to taste

For the Zoodles:
- 4 medium zucchinis
- 2 tablespoons olive oil
- 2 cloves garlic, minced
- Salt and black pepper to taste

For Serving:
- 1 cup marinara sauce (sugar-free or homemade)
- Fresh basil leaves (for garnish, optional)

Instructions:

1. **Prepare the Meatballs:** Preheat your oven to 375°F (190°C). Line a baking sheet with parchment paper. In a large bowl, combine ground turkey, Parmesan cheese, parsley, onion, egg, minced garlic, oregano, basil, salt, and black pepper. Mix until well combined. Form the mixture into 1-inch meatballs and place them on the prepared baking sheet. Bake in the preheated oven for 20-25 minutes, or until the meatballs are cooked through and have an internal temperature of 165°F (74°C).
2. **Prepare the Zoodles:** While the meatballs are baking, use a spiralizer or julienne peeler to make zucchini noodles (zoodles). Heat olive oil in a large skillet over medium heat. Add minced garlic and cook for about 1 minute, or until fragrant. Add the zoodles to the skillet and cook for 3-4 minutes, stirring occasionally, until the zoodles are tender but still crisp. Season with salt and black pepper to taste.
3. **Serve:** Toss the cooked zoodles with marinara sauce in the skillet, if desired, or serve the sauce on the side. Arrange the turkey meatballs on a plate and serve alongside the zoodles. Garnish with fresh basil leaves if desired.

Nutrients (per serving)

Calories: 300 Sodium: 450 mg Carbohydrates: 10 g
Fiber: 3 g Protein: 28 g Calcium: 150 mg Fat: 15 g
Sugar: 5 g

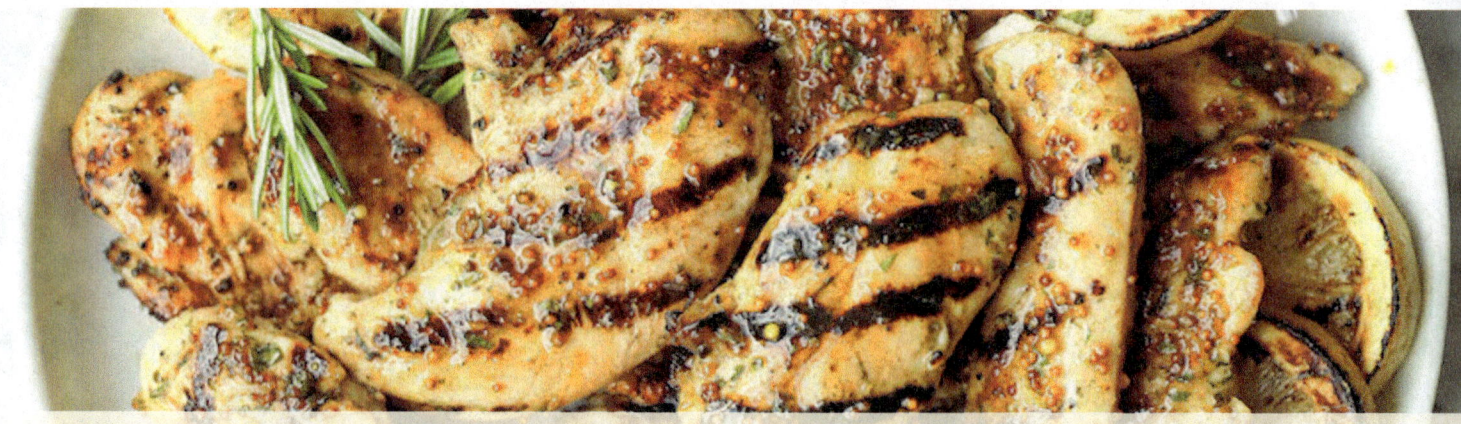

HONEY MUSTARD GRILLED CHICKEN

Honey Mustard Grilled Chicken is a delicious and easy-to-make dish that features juicy chicken breasts marinated in a tangy-sweet honey mustard sauce. Perfect for a weeknight dinner or a summer barbecue, this recipe combines simple ingredients for a flavorful, crowd-pleasing meal.

Serves 	Preparation Time	Cooking Time 
4	10 minutes	16 minute

Ingredients:

- 4 boneless, skinless chicken breasts
- 1/4 cup Dijon mustard
- 2 tablespoons honey
- 2 tablespoons olive oil
- 2 tablespoons apple cider vinegar
- 2 cloves garlic, minced
- 1 teaspoon dried thyme
- 1 teaspoon dried rosemary
- Salt and black pepper to taste

Instructions:

1. **Prepare the Marinade:** In a bowl, whisk together Dijon mustard, honey, olive oil, apple cider vinegar, minced garlic, dried thyme, dried rosemary, salt, and black pepper.
2. **Marinate the Chicken:** Place the chicken breasts in a resealable plastic bag or shallow dish. Pour the marinade over the chicken, ensuring all pieces are well coated. Seal the bag or cover the dish and refrigerate for at least 30 minutes, or up to 4 hours for more flavor.
3. **Grill the Chicken:** Preheat your grill to medium-high heat. Lightly oil the grill grates. Remove the chicken from the marinade, letting any excess drip off. Discard the remaining marinade. Grill the chicken for 6-8 minutes per side, or until the chicken reaches an internal temperature of 165°F (74°C) and has nice grill marks.
4. **Serve:** Remove the chicken from the grill and let it rest for a few minutes before slicing. Serve with your favorite side dishes or a fresh salad.

Nutrients (per serving)

Calories: 250 Sodium: 150 mg Carbohydrates: 10 g
Fiber: 0 g Protein: 30 g Calcium: 15 mg Fat: 12 g
Sugar: 9 g

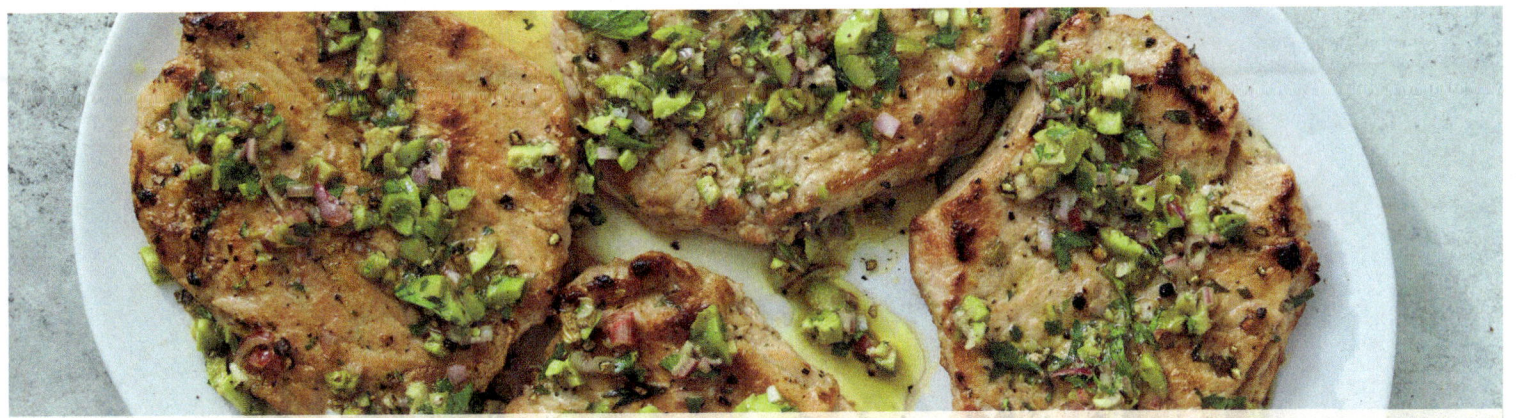

GARLIC AND HERB GRILLED PORK CHOPS

Garlic and Herb Grilled Pork Chops are a flavorful and easy-to-make dish perfect for grilling season. The savory combination of garlic, herbs, and spices creates a deliciously juicy and tender pork chop that's sure to be a hit at any barbecue or family dinner.

Serves	Preparation Time	Cooking Time
4	10 minutes	15 minute

Ingredients:

4 bone-in or boneless pork chops (about 1 inch thick)
3 tablespoons olive oil
4 cloves garlic, minced
1 tablespoon fresh rosemary, chopped (or 1 teaspoon dried)
1 tablespoon fresh thyme, chopped (or 1 teaspoon dried)
1 teaspoon paprika
1 teaspoon onion powder
Salt and black pepper to taste

Instructions:

1. **Prepare the Marinade:** In a small bowl, combine olive oil, minced garlic, rosemary, thyme, paprika, onion powder, salt, and black pepper. Mix well.
2. **Marinate the Pork Chops:** Rub the garlic and herb mixture evenly over both sides of the pork chops. Place the pork chops in a resealable plastic bag or shallow dish. Cover and refrigerate for at least 30 minutes, or up to 4 hours for more flavor.
3. **Grill the Pork Chops:** Preheat your grill to medium-high heat. Lightly oil the grill grates. Remove the pork chops from the marinade, letting any excess drip off. Discard the remaining marinade. Grill the pork chops for 6-8 minutes per side, or until they reach an internal temperature of 145°F (63°C) and have nice grill marks.
4. **Serve:** Remove the pork chops from the grill and let them rest for 5 minutes before serving. Serve with your favorite sides or a fresh salad.

Nutrients (per serving)

Calories: 290 Sodium: 180 mg Carbohydrates: 1 g
Fiber: 0 g Protein: 28 g Calcium: 20 mg Fat: 19 g
Sugar: 0 g

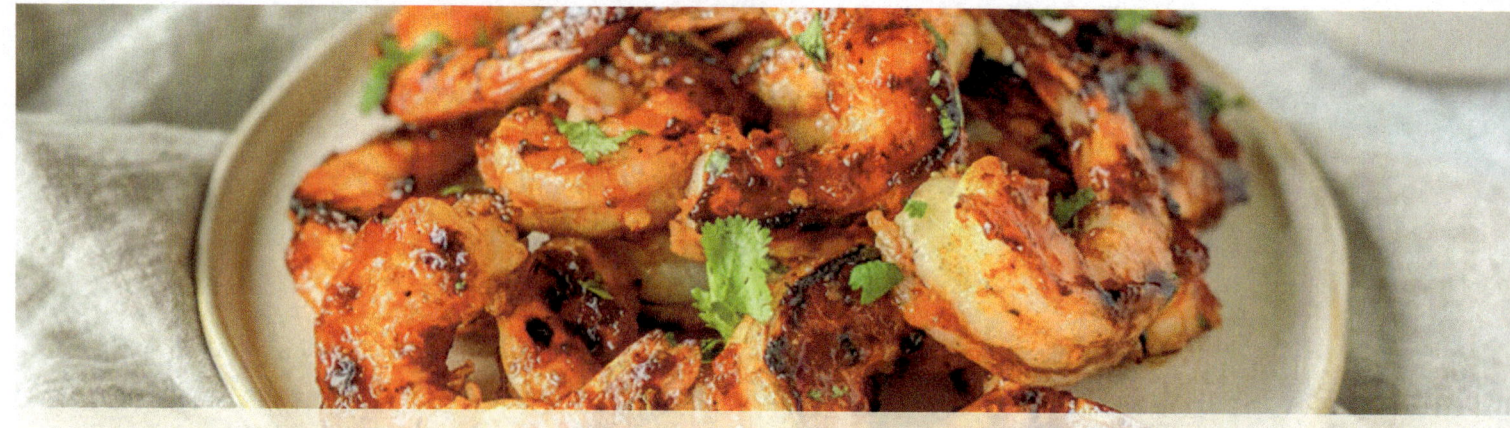

SPICY GRILLED SHRIMP SKEWERS

Spicy Grilled Shrimp Skewers offer a burst of flavor with every bite, featuring succulent shrimp marinated in a spicy, zesty sauce. Perfect for a quick and easy meal, these skewers are ideal for grilling season and can be served as an appetizer or a main course.

Serves	Preparation Time	Cooking Time 
4	15 minutes	8 minute

Ingredients:

- 1 pound large shrimp, peeled and deveined
- 2 tablespoons olive oil
- 2 tablespoons lemon juice
- 2 cloves garlic, minced
- 1 teaspoon paprika
- 1 teaspoon cayenne pepper (adjust to taste)
- 1 teaspoon ground cumin
- 1/2 teaspoon salt
- 1/4 teaspoon black pepper
- Fresh parsley for garnish (optional)
- Lemon wedges for serving

Instructions:

1. **Prepare the Marinade:** In a large bowl, combine olive oil, lemon juice, minced garlic, paprika, cayenne pepper, ground cumin, salt, and black pepper. Mix well to create the marinade.
2. **Marinate the Shrimp:** Add the shrimp to the marinade, ensuring they are evenly coated. Cover the bowl and refrigerate for at least 20-30 minutes to allow the flavors to develop.
3. **Prepare the Skewers:** If using wooden skewers, soak them in water for 15-20 minutes to prevent burning. Thread the marinated shrimp onto the skewers, piercing each shrimp twice to secure it.
4. **Grill the Shrimp:** Preheat the grill to medium-high heat. Grill the shrimp skewers for 2-3 minutes per side, or until the shrimp are pink and opaque, with slight char marks.
5. **Serve:** Remove the shrimp skewers from the grill and garnish with fresh parsley if desired. Serve hot with lemon wedges on the side for an extra burst of freshness.

Nutrients (per serving)

Calories: 150 Sodium: 200 mg Carbohydrates: 2 g Fiber: 0 g Protein: 25 g Calcium: 50 mg Fat: 6 g Sugar: 0 g

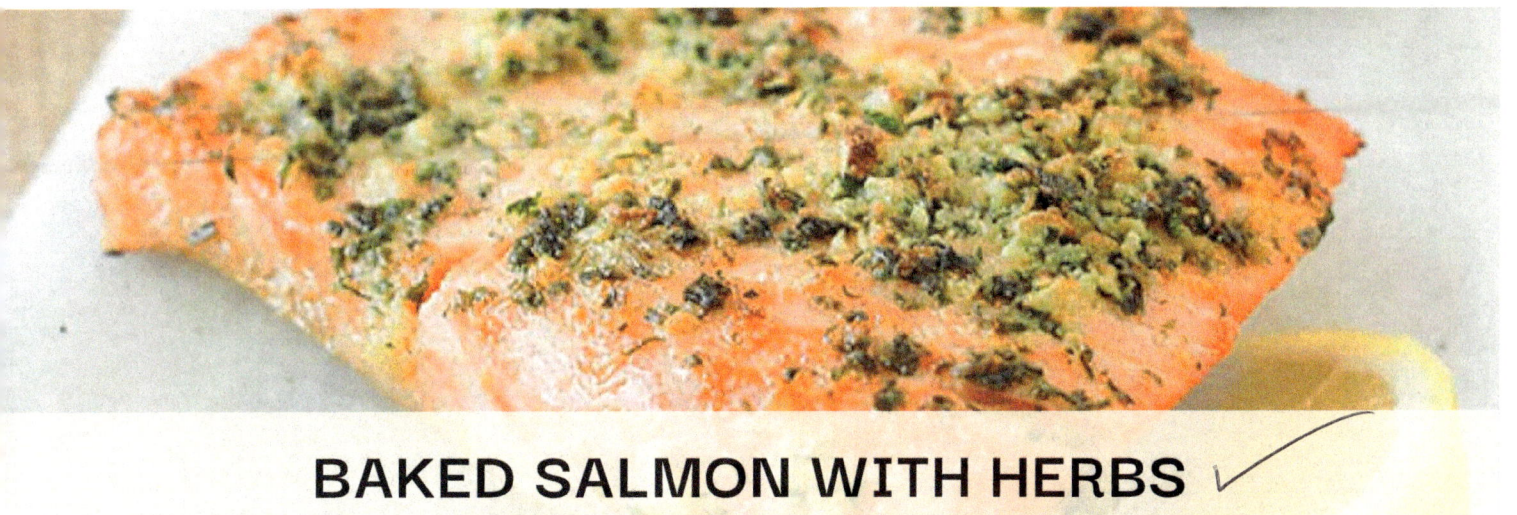

BAKED SALMON WITH HERBS ✓

Baked Salmon with Herbs is a simple yet elegant dish that's packed with flavor. The combination of fresh herbs, lemon, and garlic enhances the natural richness of the salmon, making it a perfect meal for any occasion.

Serves 	Preparation Time	Cooking Time 
4	10 minutes	15 minute

Ingredients: *½ for 2.*

- 4 salmon fillets (about 6 ounces each)
- 2 tablespoons olive oil
- 2 <u>cloves garlic, minced</u>
- 1 tablespoon fresh lemon juice
- 1 tablespoon fresh rosemary, chopped
- 1 tablespoon fresh thyme, chopped
- 1 tablespoon fresh parsley, chopped
- Salt and black pepper to taste
- Lemon slices (for garnish, optional)

Instructions:

1. **Preheat the Oven:** Preheat your oven to 400°F (200°C). Line a baking sheet with parchment paper or lightly grease it.
2. **Prepare the Herb Mixture:** In a small bowl, mix together olive oil, minced garlic, lemon juice, rosemary, thyme, parsley, salt, and black pepper.
3. **Season the Salmon:** Place the salmon fillets on the prepared baking sheet. Spoon the herb mixture evenly over the salmon fillets, making sure each piece is well-coated.
4. **Bake the Salmon:** Bake in the preheated oven for 12-15 minutes, or until the salmon flakes easily with a fork. The internal temperature of the salmon should reach 145°F (63°C).
5. **Serve:** Remove the salmon from the oven and let it rest for a few minutes. Garnish with lemon slices if desired, and serve with your favorite side dishes.

A/f. 15m.

Nutrients (per serving)

Calories: 300 Sodium: 70 mg Carbohydrates: 1 g
Fiber: 0 g Protein: 35 g Calcium: 25 mg Fat: 18 g
Sugar: 0 g

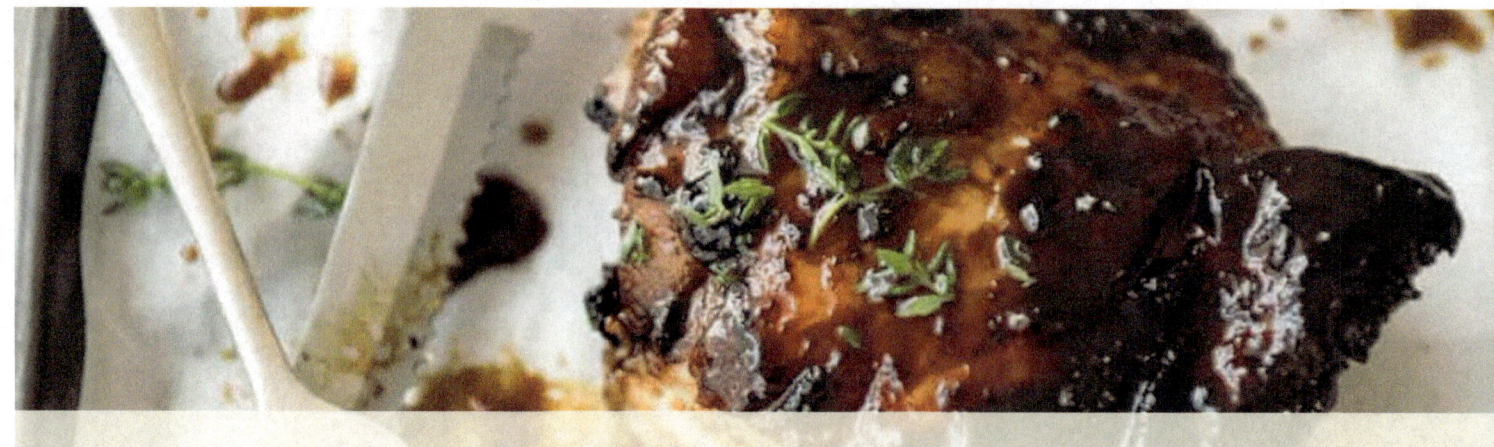

BALSAMIC GLAZED CHICKEN

Balsamic Glazed Chicken is a delightful dish where tender chicken breasts are coated in a rich, tangy balsamic reduction. This simple yet flavorful meal is perfect for a quick weeknight dinner or an elegant weekend feast.

Serves	Preparation Time	Cooking Time 
4	10 minutes	20 minute

Ingredients:

- 4 boneless, skinless chicken breasts
- 2 tablespoons olive oil
- 1/2 cup balsamic vinegar
- 2 tablespoons honey
- 2 cloves garlic, minced
- 1 teaspoon Dijon mustard
- Salt and black pepper to taste
- Fresh thyme or basil for garnish (optional)

Instructions:

1. **Prepare the Chicken:** Season the chicken breasts with salt and black pepper on both sides.
2. **Cook the Chicken:** Heat olive oil in a large skillet over medium-high heat. Add the chicken breasts and cook for about 5-7 minutes on each side, until browned and cooked through. The internal temperature should reach 165°F (74°C). Remove the chicken from the skillet and set aside.
3. **Make the Balsamic Glaze:** In the same skillet, add minced garlic and sauté for about 1 minute until fragrant. Pour in the balsamic vinegar, honey, and Dijon mustard, stirring well to combine. Allow the mixture to simmer and reduce until it thickens into a glaze, about 5-7 minutes.
4. **Glaze the Chicken:** Return the cooked chicken breasts to the skillet, spooning the balsamic glaze over each piece. Continue to cook for another 2-3 minutes, turning the chicken to ensure it's well-coated with the glaze.
5. **Serve:** Transfer the glazed chicken to a serving plate. Garnish with fresh thyme or basil if desired, and serve with your choice of side dishes.

Nutrients (per serving)

Calories: 260 Sodium: 150 mg Carbohydrates: 10 g
Fiber: 0 g Protein: 28 g Calcium: 20 mg Fat: 12 g
Sugar: 8 g

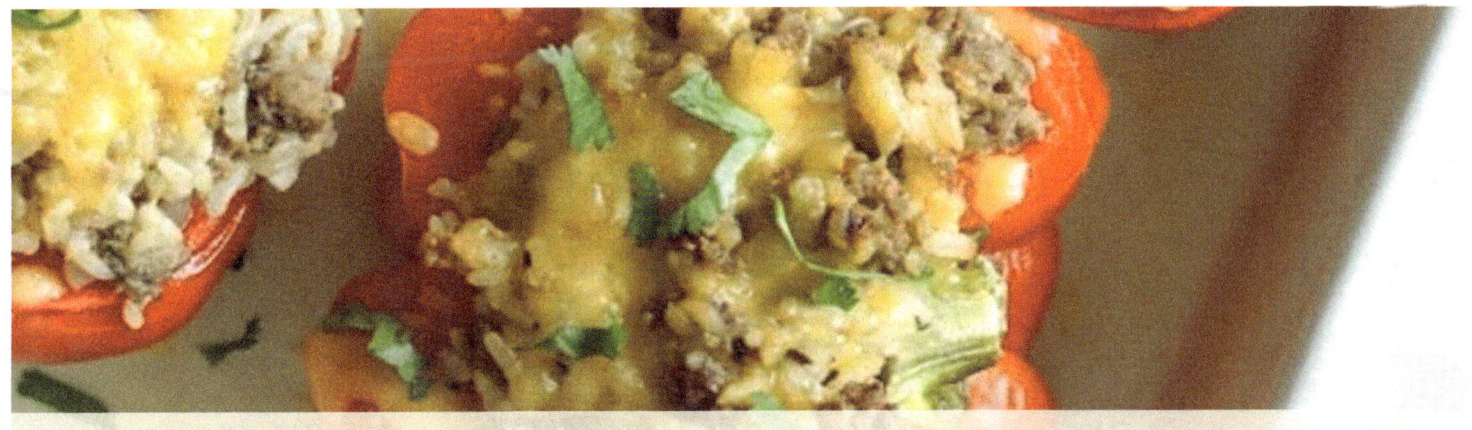

TURKEY STUFFED BELL PEPPERS

Turkey Stuffed Bell Peppers are a nutritious and delicious meal that combines lean ground turkey with vibrant bell peppers. This dish is a perfect way to enjoy a well-balanced, colorful dinner packed with protein and vegetables.

Serves	Preparation Time	Cooking Time
4	15 minutes	40 minute

Ingredients:

- 4 large bell peppers (any color)
- 1 pound ground turkey
- 1 small onion, diced
- 2 cloves garlic, minced
- 1 cup cooked quinoa or brown rice
- 1 can (14.5 oz) diced tomatoes, drained
- 1 teaspoon ground cumin
- 1 teaspoon paprika
- 1/2 teaspoon dried oregano
- Salt and black pepper to taste
- 1/2 cup shredded cheese (optional)
- Fresh parsley or cilantro for garnish

Instructions:

1. **Prepare the Bell Peppers:** Preheat your oven to 375°F (190°C). Cut the tops off the bell peppers and remove the seeds and membranes. Lightly grease a baking dish and place the peppers cut-side up in the dish.
2. **Cook the Turkey Filling:** Heat a large skillet over medium heat. Add the diced onion and cook until softened, about 3 minutes. Add the minced garlic and cook for another minute until fragrant. Add the ground turkey to the skillet, breaking it up with a spoon, and cook until browned and cooked through, about 6-8 minutes. Stir in the cooked quinoa or brown rice, drained diced tomatoes, ground cumin, paprika, oregano, salt, and black pepper. Mix well to combine and let it cook for another 2-3 minutes to blend the flavors.
3. **Stuff the Peppers:** Spoon the turkey mixture evenly into the prepared bell peppers, pressing the filling down gently. If using cheese, sprinkle the shredded cheese on top of each stuffed pepper.
4. **Bake the Peppers:** Cover the baking dish with aluminum foil and bake in the preheated oven for 25-30 minutes, until the peppers are tender. If desired, remove the foil for the last 5 minutes to let the cheese brown slightly.
5. **Serve:** Remove the stuffed bell peppers from the oven and let them cool slightly. Garnish with fresh parsley or cilantro and serve warm.

Nutrients (per serving)

Calories: 320 Sodium: 450 mg Carbohydrates: 18 g
Fiber: 4 g Protein: 29 g Calcium: 60 mg Fat: 14 g
Sugar: 6 g

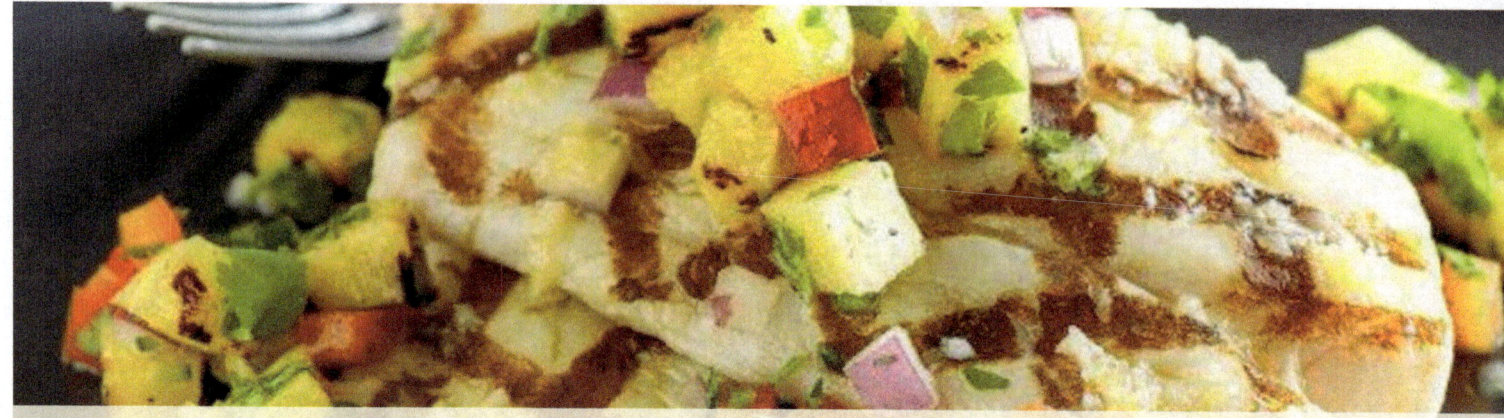

GRILLED MAHI MAHI WITH PINEAPPLE SALSA

Grilled Mahi Mahi with Pineapple Salsa is a tropical delight that pairs tender, flaky fish with a vibrant, sweet, and tangy salsa. This dish is light, refreshing, and perfect for a healthy weeknight dinner or a special weekend meal.

Serves	Preparation Time	Cooking Time 
4	15 minutes	10 minute

Ingredients:

4 Mahi Mahi fillets (about 6 oz each)
2 tablespoons olive oil
1 teaspoon garlic powder
1 teaspoon onion powder
1 teaspoon paprika
1/2 teaspoon ground cumin
Salt and black pepper to taste
1 lime, cut into wedges

For the Pineapple Salsa:
1 cup fresh pineapple, diced
1/2 red bell pepper, diced
1/4 red onion, finely chopped
1 small jalapeño, seeded and finely chopped
2 tablespoons fresh cilantro, chopped
Juice of 1 lime
Salt to taste

Instructions:

1. **Prepare the Pineapple Salsa:** In a medium bowl, combine the diced pineapple, red bell pepper, red onion, jalapeño, cilantro, and lime juice. Season with salt to taste, then mix well. Set aside to allow the flavors to meld.
2. **Season the Mahi Mahi:** In a small bowl, mix together the olive oil, garlic powder, onion powder, paprika, cumin, salt, and black pepper. Brush the Mahi Mahi fillets with the seasoned olive oil mixture, ensuring they are evenly coated on both sides.
3. **Grill the Mahi Mahi:** Preheat your grill to medium-high heat (about 400°F or 200°C). Place the seasoned Mahi Mahi fillets on the grill and cook for 4-5 minutes per side, or until the fish is opaque and flakes easily with a fork.
4. **Serve:** Transfer the grilled Mahi Mahi to serving plates. Top each fillet with a generous spoonful of the pineapple salsa. Serve with lime wedges on the side for an extra burst of citrus flavor.

Nutrients (per serving)

Calories: 290 Sodium: 190 mg Carbohydrates: 12 g
Fiber: 2 g Protein: 35 g Calcium: 40 mg Fat: 10 g
Sugar: 8 g

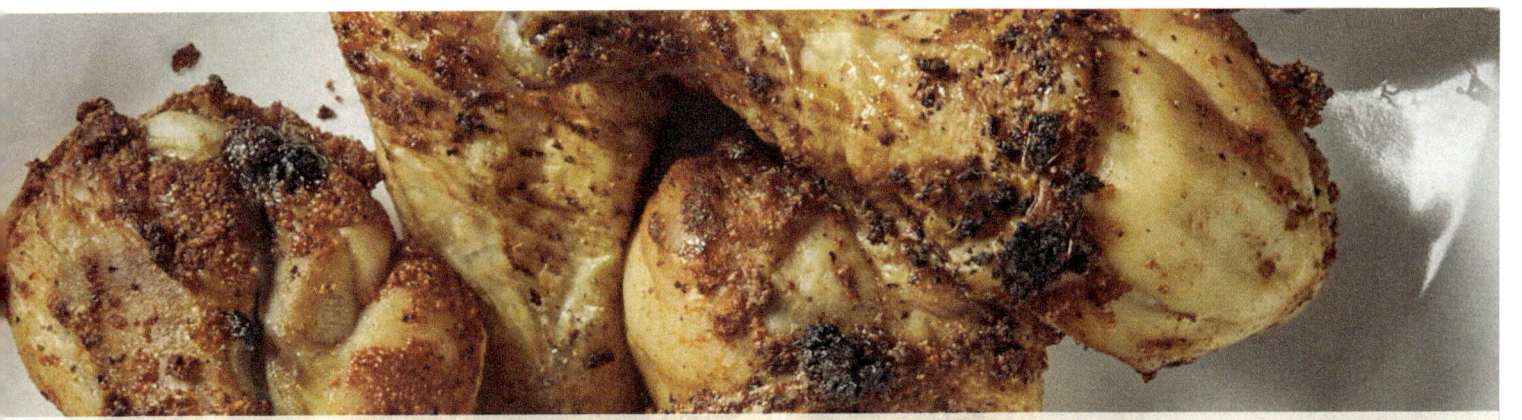

BAKED CHICKEN DRUMSTICKS

Baked Chicken Drumsticks are a simple yet flavorful dish that combines tender, juicy chicken with a crisp, seasoned exterior. This easy-to-make recipe is perfect for a weeknight dinner or meal prep, delivering delicious results with minimal effort.

Serves	Preparation Time	Cooking Time 
4	10 minutes	45 minute

Ingredients:

8 chicken drumsticks
2 tablespoons olive oil
1 teaspoon garlic powder
1 teaspoon onion powder
1 teaspoon smoked paprika
1 teaspoon dried thyme
1/2 teaspoon dried rosemary
Salt and black pepper to taste

Instructions:

1. **Preheat the Oven:** Preheat your oven to 400°F (200°C).
2. **Prepare the Drumsticks:** Pat the chicken drumsticks dry with paper towels. This helps to ensure a crispy skin. In a large bowl, combine olive oil, garlic powder, onion powder, smoked paprika, dried thyme, dried rosemary, salt, and black pepper. Toss the drumsticks in the olive oil mixture until they are evenly coated.
3. **Bake the Drumsticks:** Place the coated drumsticks on a baking sheet lined with parchment paper or aluminum foil. Arrange them in a single layer for even cooking. Bake in the preheated oven for 35-45 minutes, or until the drumsticks are golden brown and the internal temperature reaches 165°F (74°C). You can check the temperature using a meat thermometer inserted into the thickest part of the drumstick.
4. **Serve:** Remove the drumsticks from the oven and let them rest for a few minutes before serving. This helps the juices redistribute throughout the meat. Serve warm with your favorite side dishes or salads.

Nutrients (per serving)

Calories: 320 Sodium: 220 mg Carbohydrates: 0 g
Fiber: 0 g Protein: 28 g Calcium: 30 mg Fat: 23 g
Sugar: 0 g

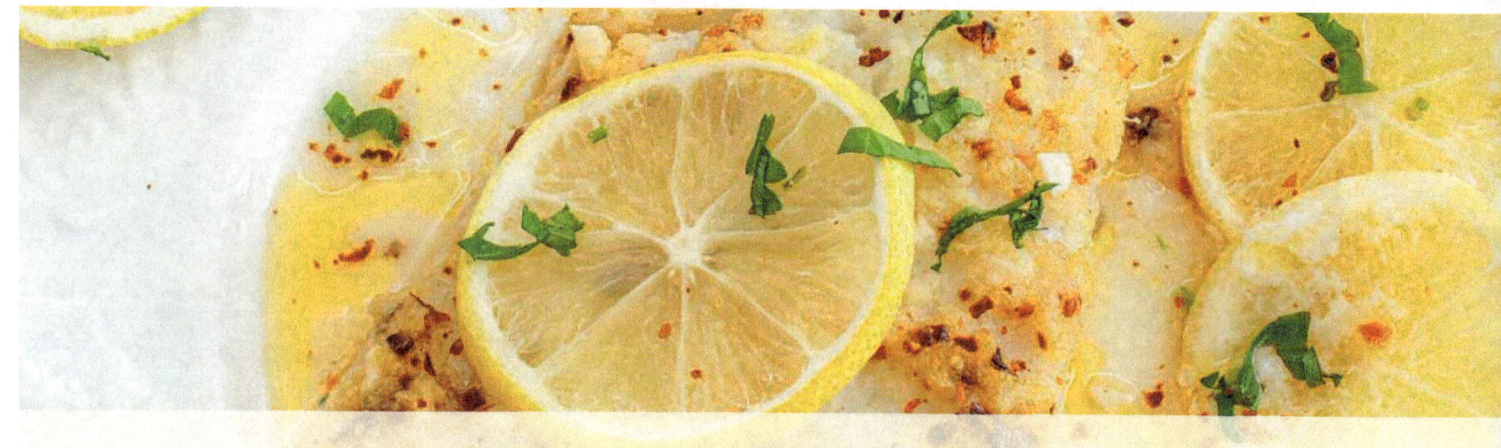

LEMON BUTTER COD

Lemon Butter Cod is a light and flavorful dish that features tender cod fillets cooked in a rich, zesty lemon butter sauce. This quick and easy recipe is perfect for a weeknight dinner or a special occasion, offering a delicious way to enjoy healthy fish.

Serves 	Preparation Time	Cooking Time 
4	10 minutes	10 minute

Ingredients:

4 cod fillets (about 6 oz each)
2 tablespoons unsalted butter
2 tablespoons olive oil
2 cloves garlic, minced
Juice and zest of 1 lemon
1 teaspoon dried parsley
Salt and black pepper to taste
Lemon wedges for serving

green veg
new spuds.

Instructions:

1. **Prepare the Cod:** Pat the cod fillets dry with paper towels and season both sides with salt and black pepper.
2. **Cook the Cod:** In a large skillet, heat the olive oil and 1 tablespoon of butter over medium-high heat. Once the butter has melted and the oil is hot, add the cod fillets. Cook for 4-5 minutes per side, or until the cod is opaque and flakes easily with a fork. Transfer the cooked fillets to a plate and cover with foil to keep warm.
3. **Make the Lemon Butter Sauce:** In the same skillet, reduce the heat to medium. Add the minced garlic and sauté for about 1 minute, until fragrant. Add the remaining 1 tablespoon of butter, lemon juice, lemon zest, and dried parsley to the skillet. Stir until the butter is melted and the sauce is well combined.
4. **Serve:** Return the cod fillets to the skillet, spooning the lemon butter sauce over the fish to coat. Serve the cod fillets with the lemon butter sauce drizzled on top and lemon wedges on the side for extra citrus flavor.

Nutrients (per serving)

Calories: 260 Sodium: 300 mg Carbohydrates: 3 g
Fiber: 0 g Protein: 30 g Calcium: 50 mg Fat: 14 g
Sugar: 1 g

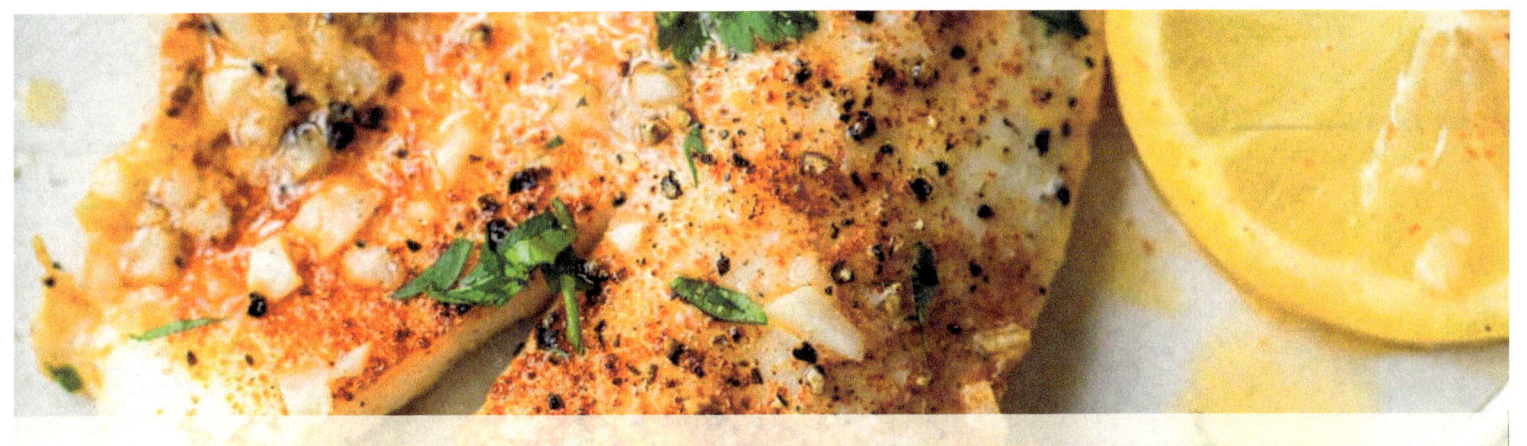

BAKED TILAPIA WITH LEMON

Baked Tilapia with Lemon is a light and flavorful dish that highlights the mild, flaky texture of tilapia. The lemon adds a bright, zesty note to the fish, making it a perfect choice for a quick and healthy meal. Ideal for both busy weeknights and leisurely dinners, this dish is easy to prepare and pairs well with a variety of sides.

Serves	Preparation Time	Cooking Time
4	10 minutes	20 minute

Ingredients:

- 4 tilapia fillets (about 6 oz each)
- 2 tablespoons olive oil
- Juice and zest of 1 lemon
- 2 cloves garlic, minced
- 1 teaspoon dried thyme
- 1 teaspoon dried oregano
- Salt and black pepper to taste
- Lemon wedges for serving
- Fresh parsley, chopped (optional, for garnish)

Instructions:

1. **Prepare the Oven and Baking Dish:** Preheat your oven to 375°F (190°C). Lightly grease a baking dish with a bit of olive oil or non-stick spray.
2. **Season the Tilapia:** Pat the tilapia fillets dry with paper towels. Place the fillets in the prepared baking dish. Drizzle the olive oil over the fillets, then sprinkle with minced garlic, dried thyme, dried oregano, salt, and black pepper. Squeeze the lemon juice over the fillets and sprinkle with lemon zest.
3. **Bake the Tilapia:** Bake the tilapia in the preheated oven for 15-20 minutes, or until the fish flakes easily with a fork and is opaque throughout. If desired, broil the fish for an additional 1-2 minutes to lightly brown the top.
4. **Serve:** Remove the tilapia from the oven and let it rest for a few minutes. Garnish with chopped fresh parsley, if using. Serve with lemon wedges on the side for an extra burst of citrus flavor.

Nutrients (per serving)

Calories: 220 Sodium: 200 mg Carbohydrates: 1 g
Fiber: 0 g Protein: 25 g Calcium: 30 mg Fat: 12 g
Sugar: 0 g

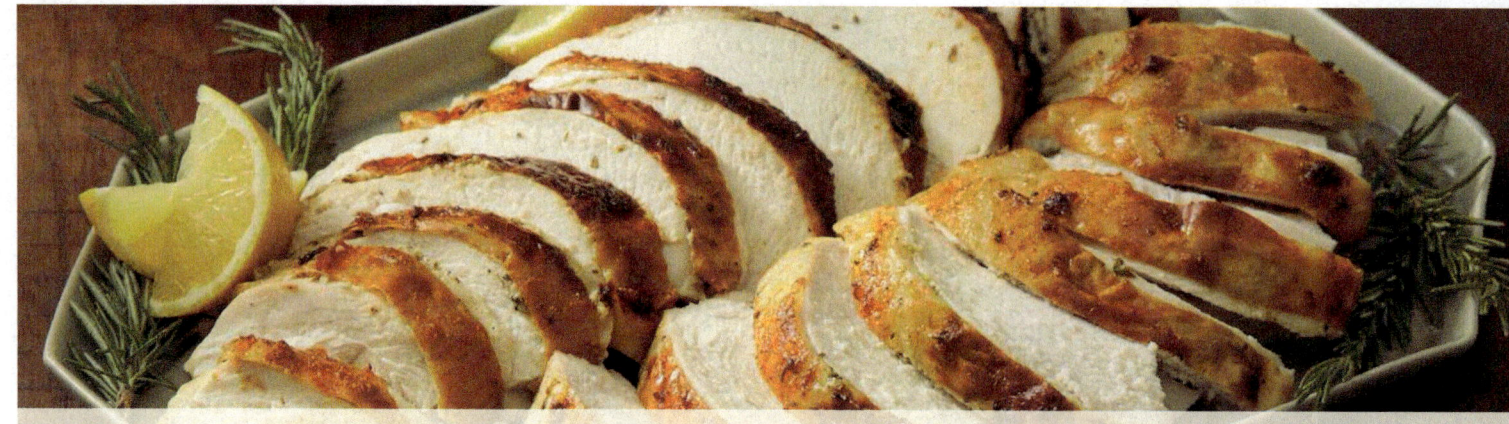

ROASTED TURKEY BREAST

Roasted Turkey Breast is a flavorful and succulent dish that's perfect for a special dinner or holiday meal. By roasting the turkey breast with a blend of herbs and spices, you get a juicy, tender result with a crispy skin. This recipe is a great option for a lean protein source and pairs well with a variety of side dishes.

Serves	 Preparation Time	Cooking Time	
4	15 minutes	1.5-2 hours	

Ingredients:

- 1 (4-5 lb) boneless, skinless turkey breast
- 2 tablespoons olive oil
- 1 tablespoon dried rosemary
- 1 tablespoon dried thyme
- 1 tablespoon garlic powder
- 1 teaspoon onion powder
- 1 teaspoon smoked paprika
- 1 teaspoon salt
- 1/2 teaspoon black pepper
- 1 cup low-sodium chicken broth
- 1 lemon, cut into wedges (for serving)
- Fresh parsley, chopped (optional, for garnish)

Instructions:

1. **Prepare the Oven and Turkey:** Preheat your oven to 375°F (190°C). Pat the turkey breast dry with paper towels. Place the turkey breast in a roasting pan.
2. **Season the Turkey:** Rub the turkey breast with olive oil. In a small bowl, combine dried rosemary, dried thyme, garlic powder, onion powder, smoked paprika, salt, and black pepper. Rub the spice mixture evenly over the turkey breast.
3. **Roast the Turkey:** Pour the chicken broth into the bottom of the roasting pan to keep the turkey moist. Roast the turkey in the preheated oven for 1.5 to 2 hours, or until the internal temperature reaches 165°F (74°C). Baste the turkey occasionally with the pan juices for extra flavor and moisture. If the skin begins to brown too quickly, cover the turkey loosely with aluminum foil.
4. **Rest and Serve:** Remove the turkey breast from the oven and let it rest for 15 minutes before slicing. This helps the juices redistribute throughout the meat. Slice the turkey breast and serve with lemon wedges and optional fresh parsley for garnish.

Nutrients (per serving)

Calories: 250 Sodium: 300 mg Carbohydrates: 1 g
Fiber: 0 g Protein: 35 g Calcium: 20 mg Fat: 10 g
Sugar: 0 g

DESSERT

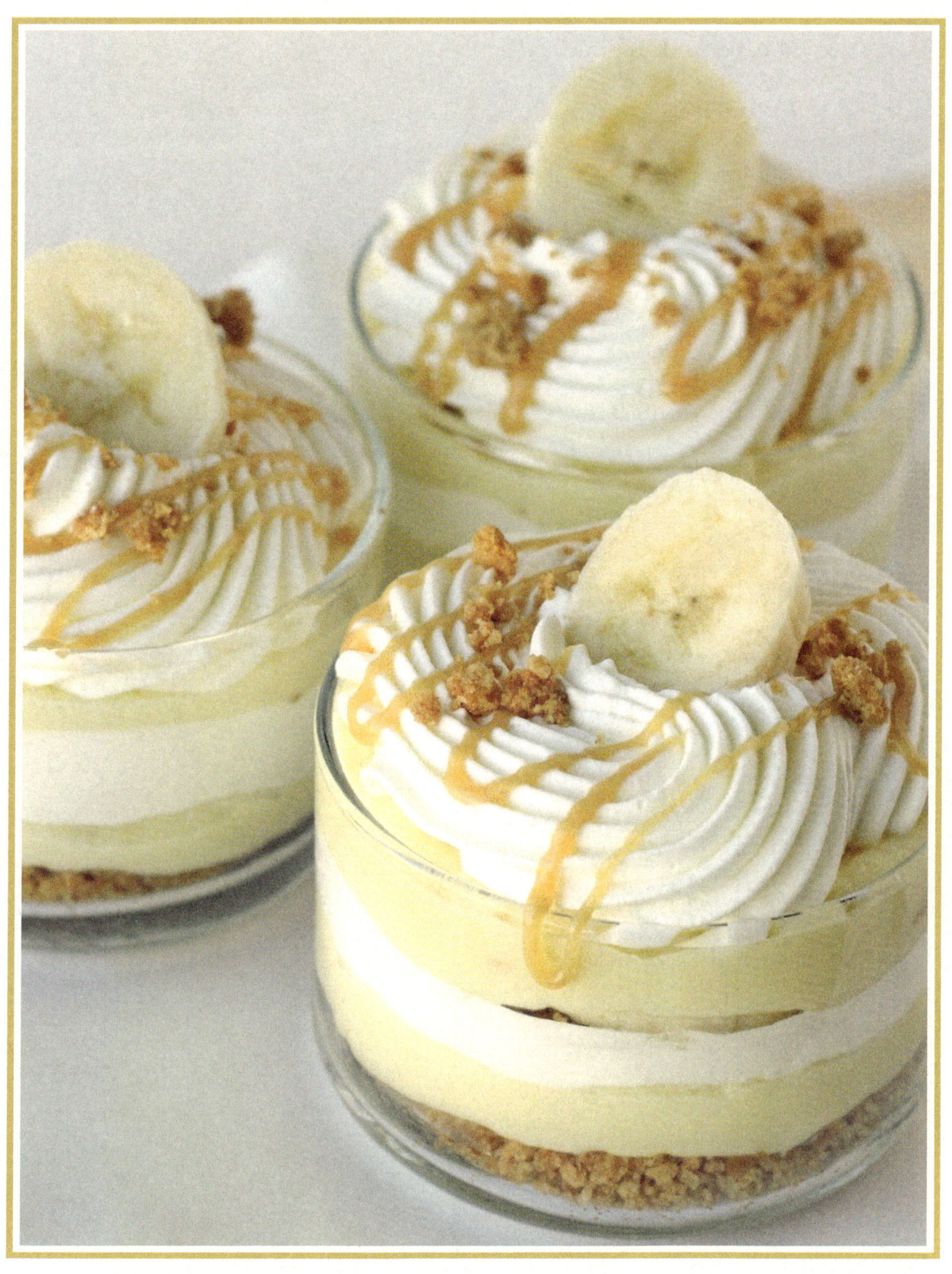

TABLE OF CONTENTS

- Chocolate Avocado Mousse (Red) — **117**
- Bacon-Wrapped Dates (Red) — **118**
- Cheesecake Bites (Red) — **119**
- Fried Mozzarella Sticks (Red) — **120**
- Buffalo Chicken Dip (Red) — **121**
- Macaroni and Cheese (Red) — **122**
- Loaded Baked Potato (Red) — **123**
- Creamy Alfredo Pasta (Red) — **124**
- Chocolate Chip Cookies (Red) — **125**
- Pecan Pie Bars (Red) — **126**
- Bacon Cheeseburger Casserole (Red) — **127**
- Chicken Alfredo Pizza (Red) — **128**
- Creamy Spinach and Artichoke Dip (Red) — **129**
- Garlic Breadsticks (Red) — **130**
- Cheddar and Broccoli Soup (Red) — **131**
- BBQ Pulled Pork Sliders (Red) — **132**
- Peanut Butter Fudge (Red) — **133**
- Caramel Popcorn (Red) — **134**
- Cheese-Stuffed Meatballs (Red) — **135**
- Fried Chicken Wings (Red) — **135**

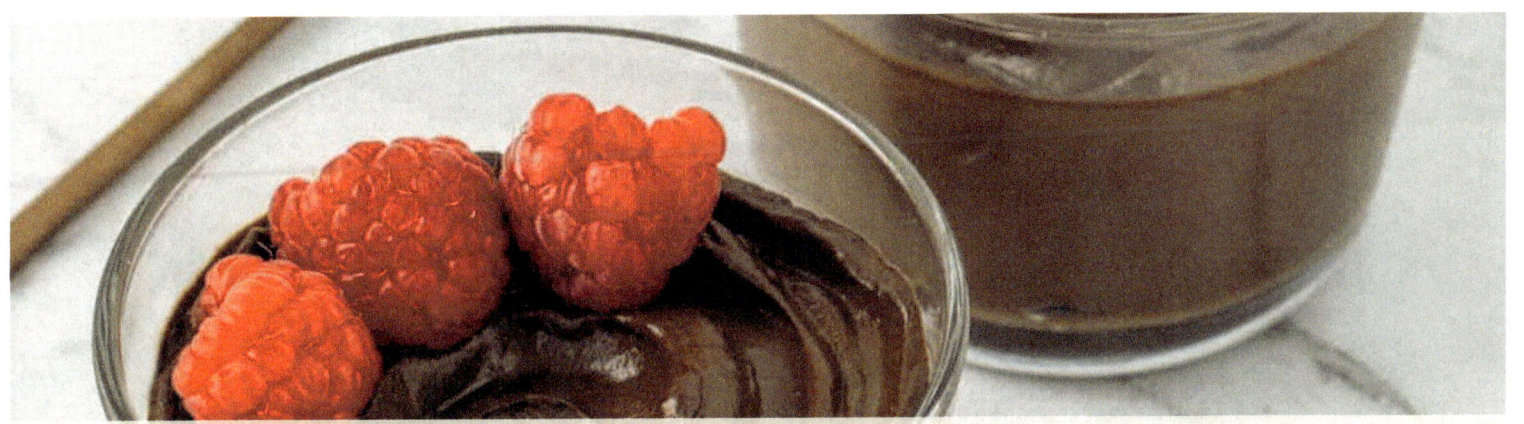

CHOCOLATE AVOCADO MOUSSE

Chocolate Avocado Mousse is a rich, creamy dessert that combines the velvety texture of avocado with the indulgent taste of chocolate. This mousse is not only delicious but also a healthier alternative to traditional chocolate mousse, as it uses avocado for a naturally smooth texture and healthy fats. Perfect for satisfying your sweet tooth while keeping things nutritious!

Serves	Preparation Time	Cooking Time	
4	10 minutes	1 hour	

Ingredients:

2 ripe avocados
1/4 cup unsweetened cocoa powder
1/4 cup pure maple syrup or honey
1/4 cup almond milk (or any milk of your choice)
1 teaspoon vanilla extract
Pinch of salt
Fresh berries or mint leaves for garnish (optional)

Instructions:

1. **Prepare the Ingredients:**
2. Cut the avocados in half, remove the pits, and scoop the flesh into a food processor or blender.
3. Add the unsweetened cocoa powder, pure maple syrup (or honey), almond milk, vanilla extract, and a pinch of salt.
4. **Blend the Mousse:**
5. Blend the ingredients until smooth and creamy. Scrape down the sides of the bowl as needed to ensure everything is well combined.
6. Taste the mousse and adjust sweetness or cocoa powder according to your preference.
7. **Chill and Serve:**
8. Transfer the mousse into serving bowls or glasses.
9. Refrigerate for at least 1 hour to allow the mousse to set and chill.
10. Garnish with fresh berries or mint leaves if desired.

Nutrients (per serving)

Calories: 180 Sodium: 10 mg Carbohydrates: 22 g
Fiber: 7 g Protein: 3 g Calcium: 50 mg Fat: 10 g
Sugar: 12 g

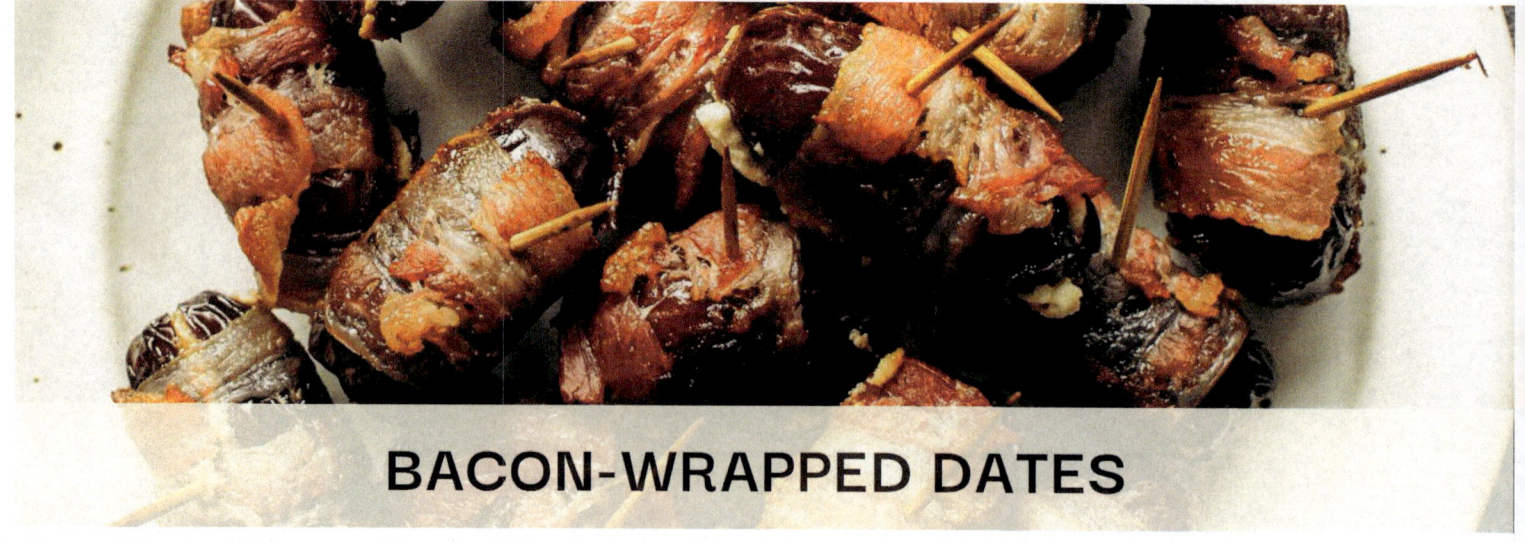

BACON-WRAPPED DATES

Bacon-Wrapped Dates are the perfect blend of sweet and savory, making them an irresistible appetizer or snack. The natural sweetness of the dates pairs wonderfully with the salty, smoky flavor of bacon, creating a bite-sized treat that's both indulgent and satisfying. Easy to prepare and even easier to enjoy, these are sure to be a hit at any gathering.

Serves	Preparation Time	Cooking Time
4	10 minutes	20 minute

Ingredients:

12 large Medjool dates, pitted
12 slices of bacon
12 whole almonds or 12 small cubes of cheese (optional)
Toothpicks

Instructions:

1. **Prepare the Dates:** Preheat your oven to 375°F (190°C). If using almonds or cheese, stuff each pitted date with one almond or a small cube of cheese.
2. **Wrap the Dates:** Cut each bacon slice in half. Wrap each date with half a slice of bacon, securing it with a toothpick to hold it in place.
3. **Bake:** Place the bacon-wrapped dates on a baking sheet lined with parchment paper or a wire rack. Bake for 15-20 minutes, turning them halfway through, until the bacon is crispy and browned.
4. **Serve:** Remove the dates from the oven and allow them to cool slightly before serving. Serve warm or at room temperature, perfect as an appetizer or snack.

Nutrients (per serving)

Calories: 180 Sodium: 10 mg Carbohydrates: 22 g
Fiber: 7 g Protein: 3 g Calcium: 50 mg Fat: 10 g
Sugar: 12 g

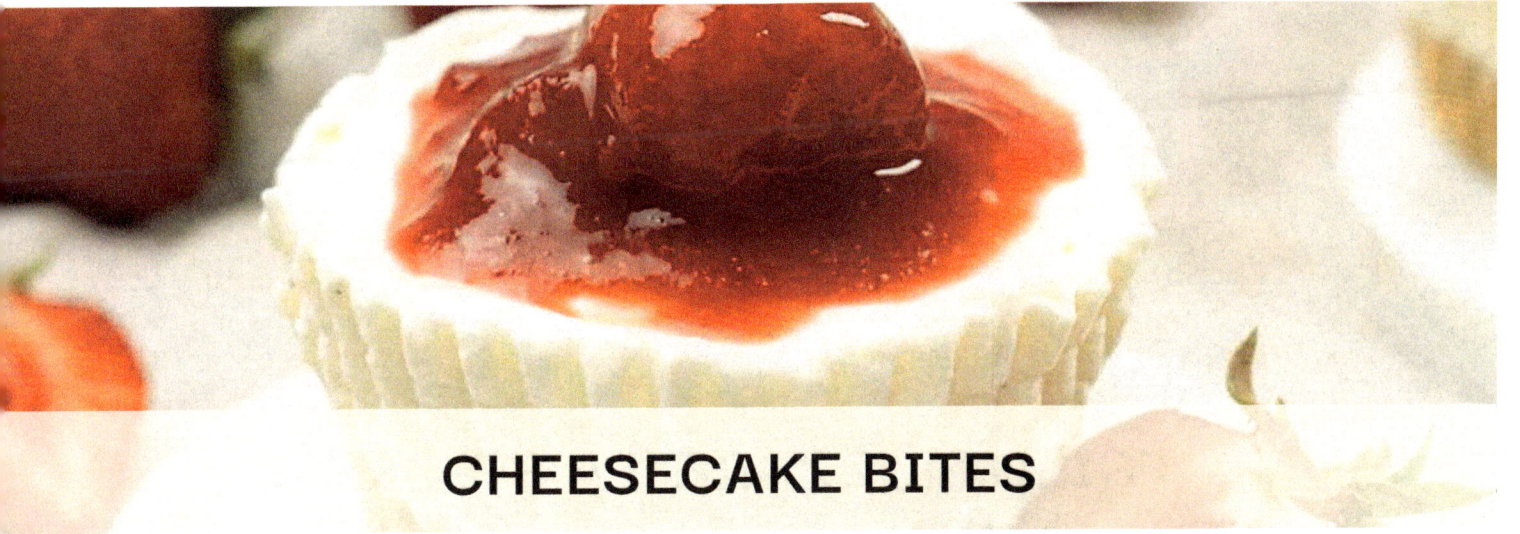

CHEESECAKE BITES

Cheesecake Bites are a delightful treat for those who love the rich, creamy taste of cheesecake but in a convenient, bite-sized form. Perfect for parties, gatherings, or just as a quick dessert, these mini cheesecakes are easy to make and even easier to enjoy. They offer all the flavor of traditional cheesecake with the added benefit of portion control.

Serves	Preparation Time	Cooking Time 
4	15 minutes	18 minute

Ingredients:

1 cup graham cracker crumbs
2 tablespoons sugar
4 tablespoons unsalted butter, melted
8 oz cream cheese, softened
1/4 cup granulated sugar
1 large egg
1 teaspoon vanilla extract
Fresh berries or fruit preserves for topping (optional)

Instructions:

1. **Prepare the Crust:** Preheat your oven to 325°F (163°C). In a small bowl, combine the graham cracker crumbs, sugar, and melted butter. Mix until the crumbs are evenly coated. Press the mixture into the bottom of a lined mini muffin tin to form the crust. Press down firmly to create an even layer.
2. **Make the Filling:** In a medium bowl, beat the softened cream cheese and sugar together until smooth and creamy. Add the egg and vanilla extract, and continue to mix until fully combined and smooth.
3. **Assemble:** Spoon the cheesecake mixture over the crust in each muffin tin, filling about 3/4 full. Smooth the tops with a spoon or spatula.
4. **Bake:** Bake in the preheated oven for 15-18 minutes, or until the edges are set and the centers are slightly jiggly. Remove from the oven and let them cool to room temperature before refrigerating for at least 2 hours to set.
5. **Serve:** Once chilled, remove the cheesecake bites from the muffin tin. Top each bite with fresh berries or a small dollop of fruit preserves if desired. Serve chilled.

Nutrients (per serving)

Calories: 80 Sodium: 50 mg Carbohydrates: 8 g
Fiber: 0 g Protein: 1 g Calcium: 15 mg Fat: 5 g
Sugar: 5 g

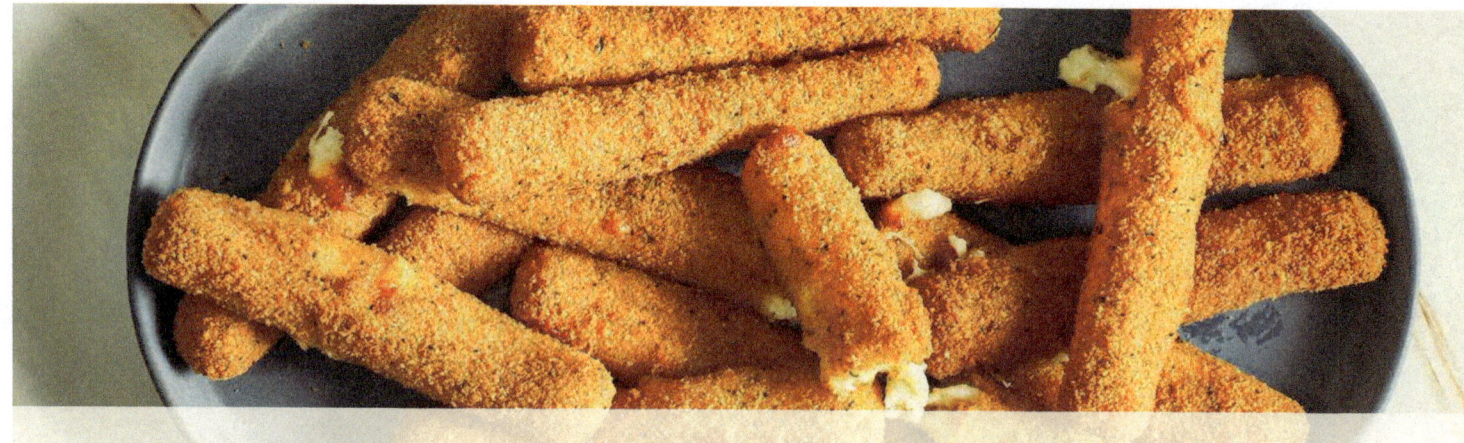

FRIED MOZZARELLA STICKS

Fried Mozzarella Sticks are a classic, crowd-pleasing appetizer that combines gooey, melted cheese with a crispy, golden-brown coating. Perfect for dipping in marinara sauce, these cheese sticks are an indulgent treat that's easy to make at home and sure to be a hit at any gathering.

Serves 	Preparation Time	Cooking Time 
4	20 minutes	10 minute

Ingredients:

12 mozzarella cheese sticks
1 cup all-purpose flour
2 large eggs
2 tablespoons water
1 1/2 cups Italian-style breadcrumbs
1/2 cup grated Parmesan cheese
1 teaspoon garlic powder
1 teaspoon dried oregano
1/2 teaspoon salt
Vegetable oil for frying
Marinara sauce for dipping

Instructions:

1. **Prepare the Cheese:** Unwrap the mozzarella sticks and cut each one in half to create 24 shorter sticks. Place the cheese sticks on a baking sheet and freeze them for at least 1 hour. This will help prevent the cheese from melting too quickly while frying.
2. **Set Up the Breading Station:** In one shallow bowl, place the flour. In a second shallow bowl, whisk together the eggs and water. In a third shallow bowl, combine the breadcrumbs, grated Parmesan cheese, garlic powder, dried oregano, and salt.
3. **Bread the Mozzarella Sticks:** Dip each frozen mozzarella stick into the flour, shaking off any excess. Then, dip it into the egg mixture, making sure it's fully coated. Finally, roll the stick in the breadcrumb mixture, pressing lightly to ensure the crumbs adhere. For an extra-crispy coating, repeat the egg and breadcrumb steps. Place the breaded mozzarella sticks back on the baking sheet and freeze them for another 30 minutes.
4. **Fry the Mozzarella Sticks:** Heat about 2 inches of vegetable oil in a large skillet or deep fryer to 350°F (175°C). Fry the mozzarella sticks in batches, about 2-3 minutes per batch, until golden brown and crispy. Avoid overcrowding the pan. Remove the fried sticks with a slotted spoon and drain them on paper towels.
5. **Serve:** Serve the fried mozzarella sticks hot with marinara sauce on the side for dipping.

Nutrients (per serving)

Calories: 90 Sodium: 150 mg Carbohydrates: 6 g
Fiber: 0 g Protein: 4 g Calcium: 100 mg Fat: 5 g
Sugar: 0 g

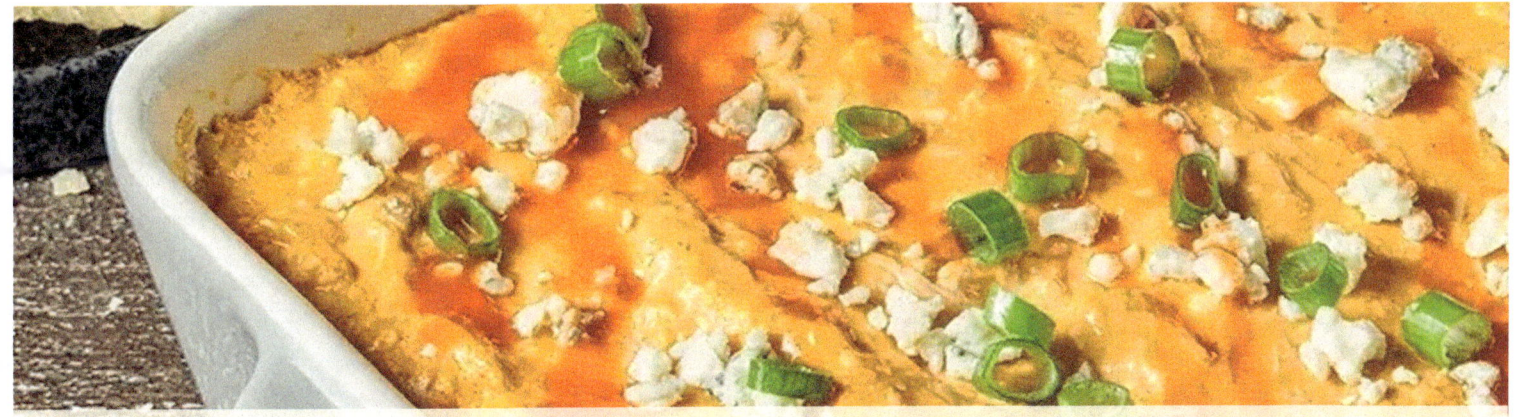

BUFFALO CHICKEN DIP

Buffalo Chicken Dip is a creamy, spicy, and flavorful appetizer that brings all the deliciousness of buffalo wings in a convenient, dippable form. Perfect for game day, parties, or any gathering, this dip pairs wonderfully with fresh veggies, crackers, or tortilla chips.

Serves	Preparation Time	Cooking Time
4	10 minutes	25 minute

Ingredients:

2 cups shredded cooked chicken (rotisserie chicken works great)
8 oz cream cheese, softened
1/2 cup ranch dressing
1/2 cup buffalo wing sauce (like Frank's RedHot)
1 cup shredded cheddar cheese
1/2 cup crumbled blue cheese (optional)
1 tablespoon chopped green onions (for garnish)
Tortilla chips, celery sticks, or carrot sticks for serving

Instructions:

1. **Preheat the Oven:** Preheat your oven to 350°F (175°C).
2. **Prepare the Dip Mixture:** In a medium mixing bowl, combine the softened cream cheese, ranch dressing, and buffalo wing sauce. Stir until smooth and well combined. Add the shredded chicken and 1/2 cup of the shredded cheddar cheese. If you like blue cheese, add the crumbled blue cheese as well. Mix until everything is evenly distributed.
3. **Bake the Dip:** Transfer the mixture to an 8x8-inch baking dish or a similar-sized oven-safe dish. Sprinkle the remaining 1/2 cup of shredded cheddar cheese over the top. Bake in the preheated oven for 20-25 minutes, or until the dip is hot and bubbly.
4. **Garnish and Serve:** Remove the dip from the oven and let it cool slightly. Garnish with chopped green onions for a pop of color and flavor. Serve the dip warm with tortilla chips, celery sticks, or carrot sticks for dipping.

Nutrients (per serving)

Calories: 200 Sodium: 600 mg Carbohydrates: 2 g
Fiber: 0 g Protein: 12 g Calcium: 100 mg Fat: 16 g
Sugar: 0 g

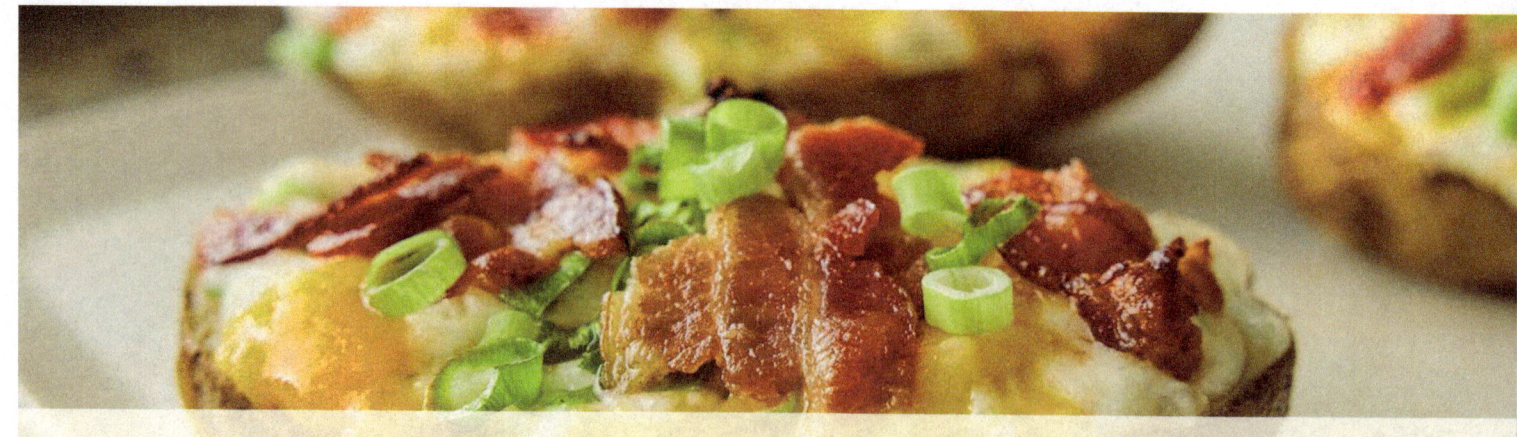

LOADED BAKED POTATO

A classic comfort food, the Loaded Baked Potato is a hearty dish that combines the creamy texture of baked potato with savory toppings like crispy bacon, melted cheese, and a dollop of sour cream. It's perfect as a side dish or even a satisfying main course.

Serves	Preparation Time	Cooking Time
4	10 minutes	60 minute

Ingredients: *for us!*

- 4 large russet potatoes — 1
- 4 slices of bacon, cooked and crumbled — 1
- 1 cup shredded cheddar cheese — 1/4
- 1/2 cup sour cream — 1/8 ✓
- 1/4 cup chopped green onions
- 2 tablespoons butter — 1/2
- Salt and pepper to taste

feta/gray/not cheddar.

Instructions: *or M/W 5m then bake (Lily!)*

1. **Preheat the Oven:** Preheat your oven to 400°F (200°C).
2. **Prepare the Potatoes:** Scrub the potatoes under running water to clean them, then dry with a towel. Poke each potato several times with a fork to allow steam to escape during baking. Rub the potatoes with a small amount of butter and sprinkle with salt for added flavor.
3. **Bake the Potatoes:** Place the prepared potatoes directly on the oven rack. Bake for 45-60 minutes, or until the potatoes are tender when pierced with a fork.
4. **Prepare the Toppings:** While the potatoes are baking, cook the bacon in a skillet over medium heat until crispy. Remove from the skillet and drain on paper towels. Once cooled, crumble the bacon. Grate the cheddar cheese, and chop the green onions.
5. **Assemble the Loaded Baked Potatoes:** Remove the baked potatoes from the oven and let them cool slightly. Carefully cut a slit lengthwise on each potato, then gently press the ends together to open up the potato. Fluff the inside of the potato with a fork and add a small pat of butter to each. Top with shredded cheddar cheese, allowing it to melt into the hot potato. Sprinkle crumbled bacon and chopped green onions over the cheese. Finish with a dollop of sour cream on top and season with salt and pepper to taste.

Nutrients (per serving)

200 Calories: ~~400~~ Sodium: 600 mg Carbohydrates: 50 g
Fiber: 5 g Protein: 14 g Calcium: 150 mg Fat: 18 g
Sugar: 2 g

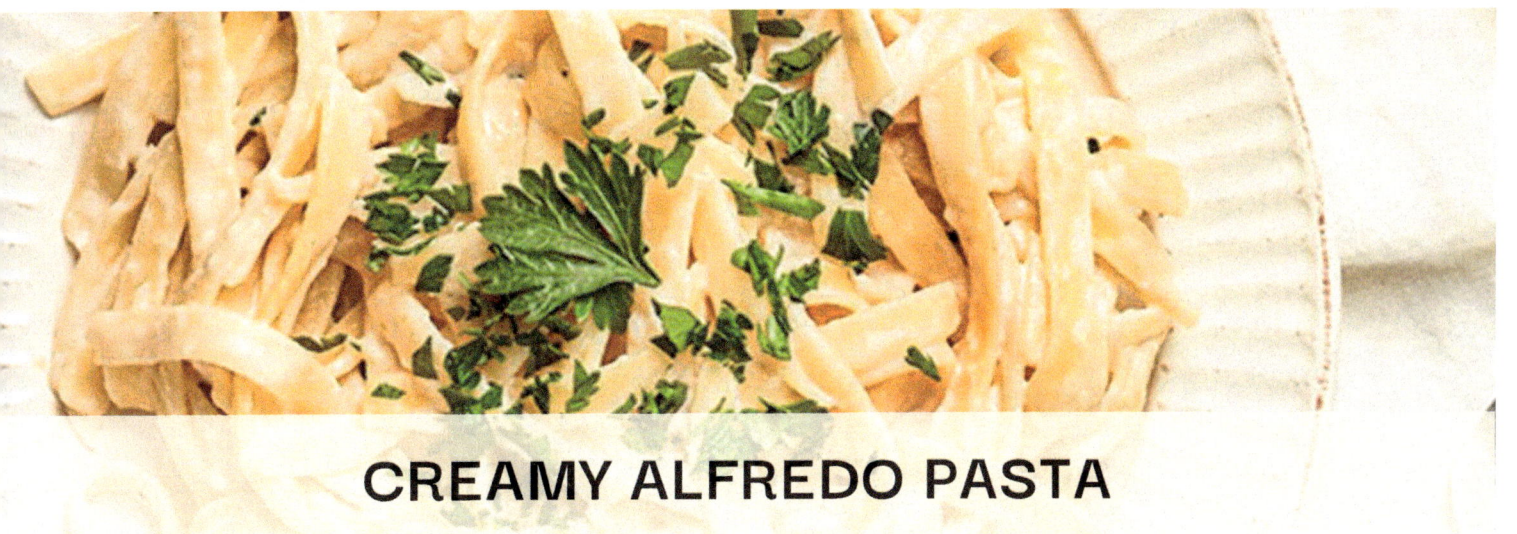

CREAMY ALFREDO PASTA

Creamy Alfredo Pasta is a rich and indulgent dish that features tender pasta coated in a luscious, velvety sauce made from butter, cream, and Parmesan cheese. It's a comforting and simple meal that can be enjoyed as a main course or paired with your favorite protein.

Serves	Preparation Time	Cooking Time 
4	10 minutes	15 minute

Ingredients:

12 oz fettuccine or your preferred pasta
1 cup heavy cream
1/2 cup unsalted butter
1 cup grated Parmesan cheese
2 cloves garlic, minced
Salt and pepper to taste
Fresh parsley, chopped (for garnish)

Instructions:

1. **Cook the Pasta:** Bring a large pot of salted water to a boil. Add the pasta and cook according to the package instructions until al dente. Drain the pasta, reserving 1/2 cup of pasta water, and set aside.
2. **Prepare the Alfredo Sauce:** In a large skillet, melt the butter over medium heat. Add the minced garlic and sauté for about 1 minute, until fragrant. Pour in the heavy cream, stirring constantly, and bring the mixture to a gentle simmer. Gradually add the grated Parmesan cheese, stirring continuously until the cheese is fully melted and the sauce is smooth. Season with salt and pepper to taste.
3. **Combine Pasta and Sauce:** Add the cooked pasta to the skillet with the Alfredo sauce, tossing to coat the pasta evenly. If the sauce is too thick, gradually add the reserved pasta water, a little at a time, until the desired consistency is reached.
4. **Serve:** Transfer the creamy Alfredo pasta to serving plates. Garnish with freshly chopped parsley and additional Parmesan cheese if desired. Serve immediately while hot.

Nutrients (per serving)

Calories: 550 Sodium: 500 mg Carbohydrates: 45 g
Fiber: 2 g Protein: 15 g Calcium: 200 mg Fat: 35 g
Sugar: 1 g

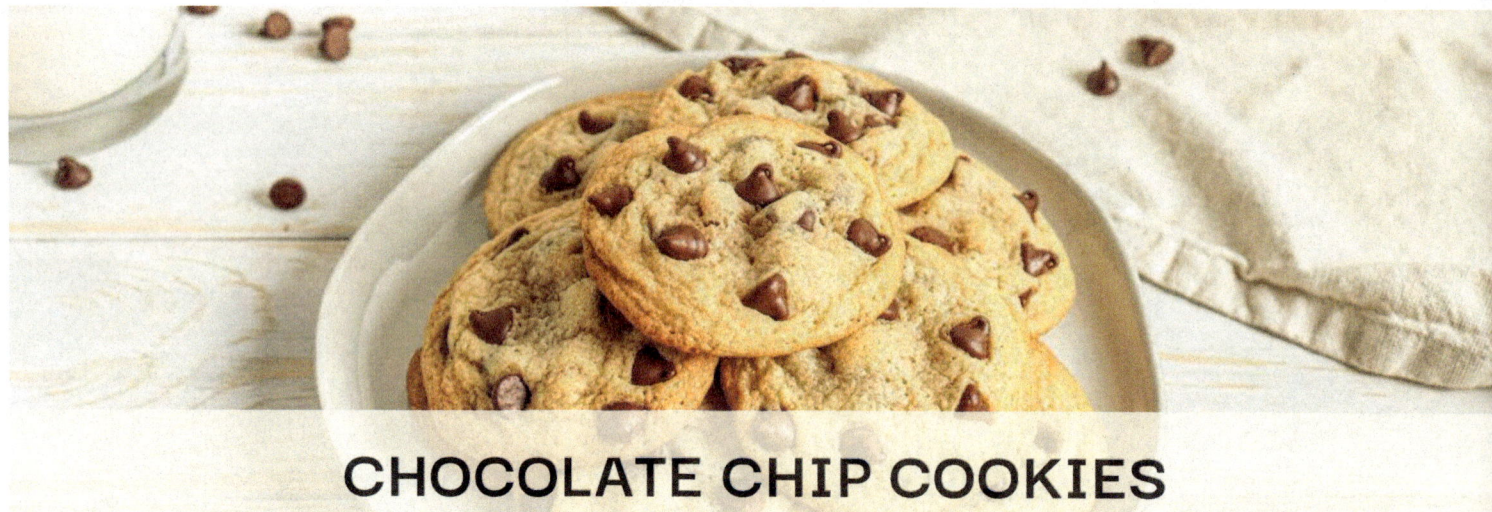

CHOCOLATE CHIP COOKIES

Chocolate Chip Cookies are a beloved classic that combines a chewy, buttery base with sweet, gooey chocolate chips. Perfect for any occasion, these cookies are a crowd-pleaser that never goes out of style.

Serves	Preparation Time 	Cooking Time 
4	15 minutes	12 minute

Ingredients:

- 1 cup (2 sticks) unsalted butter, softened
- 1 cup granulated sugar
- 1 cup packed brown sugar
- 2 large eggs
- 2 teaspoons vanilla extract
- 3 cups all-purpose flour G/F.
- 1 teaspoon baking soda
- 1/2 teaspoon baking powder
- 1/2 teaspoon salt
- 1 1/2 cups semisweet chocolate chips

Instructions:

1. **Preheat the Oven:** Preheat your oven to 350°F (175°C). Line two baking sheets with parchment paper.
2. **Prepare the Dough:** In a large bowl, cream together the softened butter, granulated sugar, and brown sugar until light and fluffy.Beat in the eggs one at a time, then mix in the vanilla extract.
3. **Mix Dry Ingredients:** In a separate bowl, whisk together the flour, baking soda, baking powder, and salt.
4. **Combine:** Gradually add the dry ingredients to the wet ingredients, mixing just until combined.Stir in the chocolate chips.
5. **Form the Cookies:** Drop rounded tablespoons of dough onto the prepared baking sheets, spacing them about 2 inches apart.
6. **Bake:** Bake in the preheated oven for 10-12 minutes, or until the edges are golden brown but the centers are still soft.Allow the cookies to cool on the baking sheets for a few minutes before transferring them to wire racks to cool completely.
7. **Serve:** Enjoy the cookies warm or at room temperature.

Nutrients (per serving)

Calories: 150 Sodium: 80 mg Carbohydrates: 22 g

Fiber: 1 g Protein: 2 g Calcium: 30 mg Fat: 8 g

Sugar: 15 g

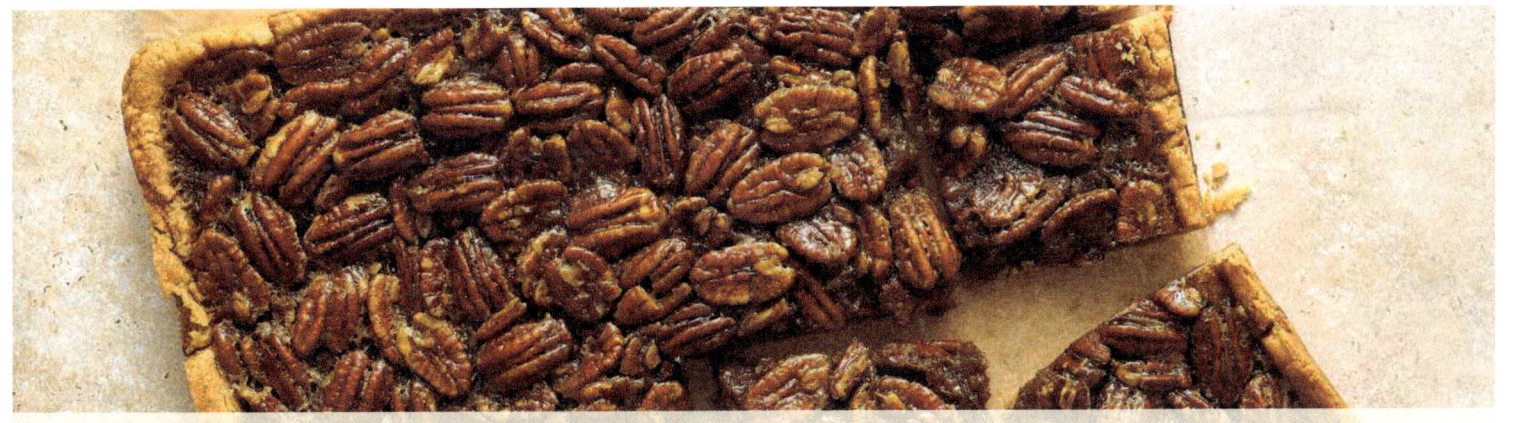

PECAN PIE BARS

Pecan Pie Bars are a delightful twist on the classic pecan pie, offering all the rich, nutty flavor of the traditional dessert in an easy-to-serve bar form. With a buttery crust and a gooey, nutty filling, these bars are perfect for holiday gatherings or as a sweet treat any time of year.

Serves	Preparation Time	Cooking Time
4	15 minutes	50 minute

Ingredients:

For the Crust:
1 1/2 cups all-purpose flour *GF*
1/2 cup granulated sugar
1/2 cup unsalted butter, cold and cut into small pieces
1/4 teaspoon salt

For the Filling:
1 cup light corn syrup *— golden syrup*
1 cup packed brown sugar
1/2 cup unsalted butter, melted
3 large eggs
1 teaspoon vanilla extract
1 1/2 cups pecan halves

Instructions:

1. **Preheat the Oven:** Preheat your oven to 350°F (175°C). Line an 8x8-inch baking pan with parchment paper, leaving a bit of an overhang for easy removal. *sling-*
2. **Prepare the Crust:** In a medium bowl, combine the flour, sugar, and salt. Cut in the cold butter using a pastry cutter or your fingers until the mixture resembles coarse crumbs. Press the mixture evenly into the bottom of the prepared baking pan.
3. **Bake the Crust:** Bake in the preheated oven for 15 minutes, or until lightly golden. Remove from the oven and set aside.
4. **Prepare the Filling:** In a large bowl, whisk together the corn syrup, brown sugar, melted butter, eggs, and vanilla extract until smooth. Stir in the pecan halves until evenly distributed.
5. **Assemble and Bake:** Pour the pecan filling over the partially baked crust, spreading it out evenly. Return to the oven and bake for an additional 30-35 minutes, or until the filling is set and the top is golden brown.
6. **Cool and Cut:** Allow the bars to cool completely in the pan on a wire rack before lifting them out using the parchment paper overhang. Once cooled, cut into squares or bars.
7. **Serve:** Serve at room temperature or chilled. Enjoy with a dollop of whipped cream or a scoop of vanilla ice cream, if desired.

Nutrients (per serving)

Calories: 250 Sodium: 100 mg Carbohydrates: 30 g
Fiber: 1 g Protein: 3 g Calcium: 20 mg Fat: 15 g
Sugar: 20 g

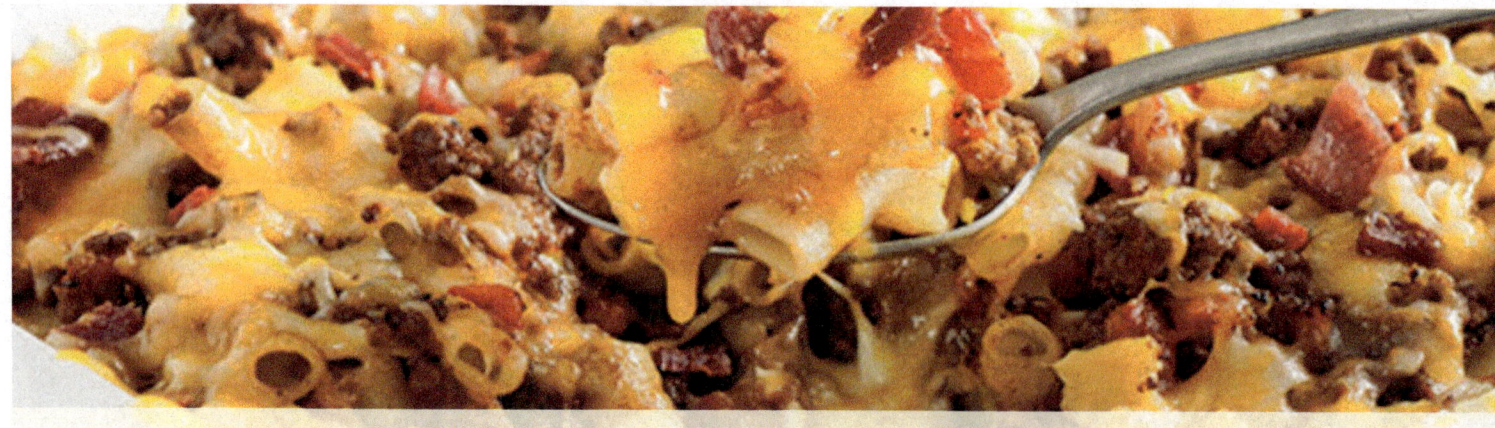

BACON CHEESEBURGER CASSEROLE

Bacon Cheeseburger Casserole is a comforting and hearty dish that combines the flavors of a classic cheeseburger with the convenience of a casserole. Packed with ground beef, crispy bacon, melted cheese, and seasoned with savory spices, this dish is perfect for a family dinner or potluck.

Serves	Preparation Time 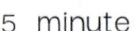	Cooking Time 
4	15 minutes	35 minute

Ingredients:

- 1 lb (450g) ground beef
- 6 slices bacon, chopped
- 1 small onion, diced
- 2 cloves garlic, minced
- 1 cup shredded cheddar cheese
- 1/2 cup shredded mozzarella cheese
- 1/4 cup ketchup
- 1 tablespoon Dijon mustard
- 1 tablespoon Worcestershire sauce
- 1 teaspoon paprika
- 1/2 teaspoon black pepper
- 1/2 teaspoon salt
- 1/2 cup mayonnaise
- 1 large egg
- 2 cups cooked cauliflower rice (for a low-carb version) or regular rice

Instructions:

1. **Preheat the Oven:** Preheat your oven to 375°F (190°C). Grease a 9x13-inch baking dish or spray with non-stick cooking spray.
2. **Cook the Bacon and Beef:** In a large skillet over medium heat, cook the chopped bacon until crispy. Remove with a slotted spoon and set aside, leaving the bacon drippings in the pan. Add the diced onion to the skillet and cook until softened, about 3 minutes. Stir in the minced garlic and cook for another 30 seconds. Add the ground beef to the skillet, breaking it up with a spoon. Cook until browned and cooked through. Drain any excess fat.
3. **Mix the Ingredients:** In a large bowl, combine the cooked beef and onion mixture with the cooked bacon, shredded cheddar cheese, shredded mozzarella cheese, ketchup, Dijon mustard, Worcestershire sauce, paprika, black pepper, and salt. Stir until well combined.
4. **Prepare the Casserole:** Stir in the mayonnaise and egg until everything is evenly mixed. Fold in the cooked cauliflower rice (or regular rice).
5. **Assemble and Bake:** Spread the mixture evenly into the prepared baking dish. Bake in the preheated oven for 25-30 minutes, or until the casserole is hot and bubbly and the cheese is melted and slightly golden.
6. **Serve:** Let the casserole cool for a few minutes before serving. Garnish with extra chopped bacon or fresh herbs if desired.

Nutrients (per serving)

Calories: 320   Sodium: 600 mg   Carbohydrates: 10 g
Fiber: 2 g   Protein: 20 g   Calcium: 150 mg   Fat: 22 g
Sugar: 6

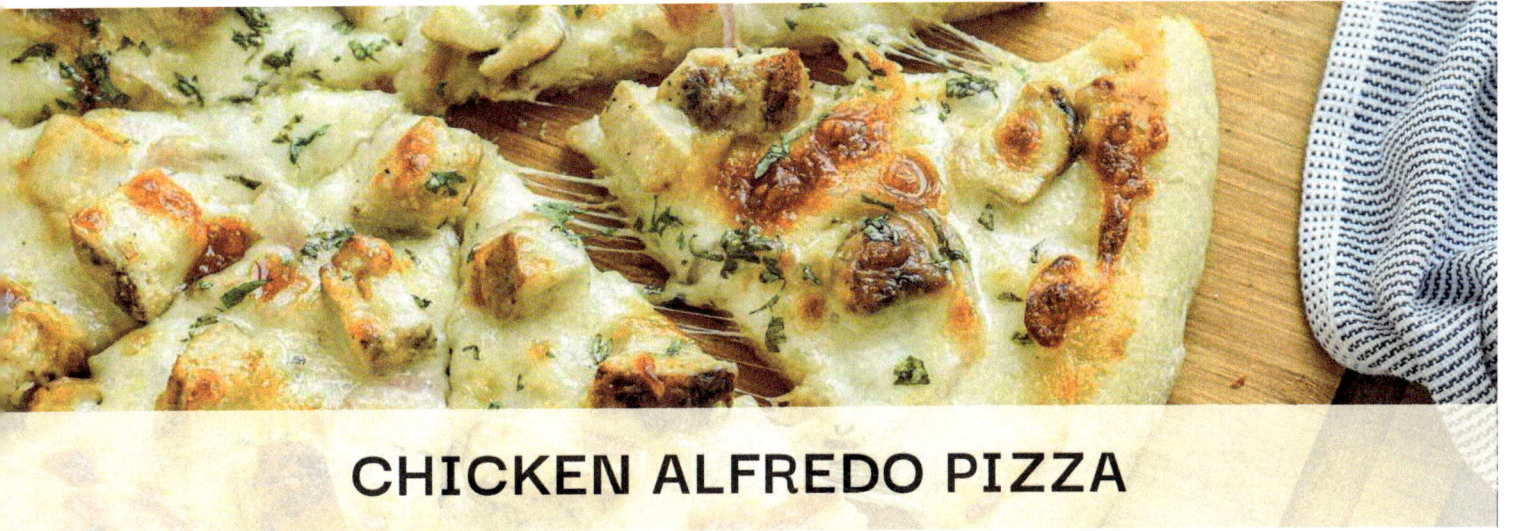

CHICKEN ALFREDO PIZZA

Chicken Alfredo Pizza is a delicious twist on traditional pizza, featuring a creamy Alfredo sauce base instead of the classic tomato sauce. Topped with tender chicken, melted mozzarella cheese, and a sprinkle of Parmesan, this pizza is rich and flavorful, making it a perfect choice for a comforting meal.

Serves	Preparation Time	Cooking Time 
4	15 minutes	15 minute

Ingredients:

For the Pizza Crust:
1 package (13.8 oz) refrigerated pizza dough or pre-made pizza crust (or use a low-carb cauliflower crust for a healthier option)

For the Alfredo Sauce:
1/2 cup heavy cream
1/4 cup unsalted butter
1/2 cup grated Parmesan cheese
2 cloves garlic, minced
1/4 teaspoon salt
1/4 teaspoon black pepper

For the Pizza Topping:
1 cup cooked chicken breast, shredded or diced
1 cup shredded mozzarella cheese
1/4 cup grated Parmesan cheese
1/2 cup sliced mushrooms
1/4 cup sliced black olives (optional)
1/4 cup chopped fresh basil or parsley (for garnish)

Instructions:

1. **Prepare the Oven and Pizza Crust:** Preheat your oven to 450°F (232°C). If using a pizza stone, place it in the oven while preheating. Roll out the pizza dough on a lightly floured surface to your desired thickness. If using a pre-made crust, follow the package instructions.
2. **Make the Alfredo Sauce:** In a small saucepan, melt the butter over medium heat. Add the minced garlic and cook for about 1 minute until fragrant. Stir in the heavy cream and bring to a simmer. Cook for 2-3 minutes, stirring frequently, until the cream is slightly thickened. Reduce the heat to low and gradually add the Parmesan cheese, stirring until melted and smooth. Season with salt and pepper. Remove from heat.
3. **Assemble the Pizza:** Spread a thin layer of the Alfredo sauce over the prepared pizza crust, leaving a small border around the edges. Evenly distribute the shredded chicken over the sauce. Sprinkle the shredded mozzarella cheese and additional Parmesan cheese over the chicken. Top with sliced mushrooms and black olives (if using).
4. **Bake the Pizza:** Transfer the pizza to the preheated oven or onto the pizza stone. Bake for 12-15 minutes, or until the crust is golden and the cheese is melted and bubbly.
5. **Serve:** Remove the pizza from the oven and let it cool for a few minutes. Garnish with chopped fresh basil or parsley before slicing and serving.

Nutrients (per serving)

Calories: 280 Sodium: 600 mg Carbohydrates: 18 g
Fiber: 1 g Protein: 15 g Calcium: 300 mg Fat: 16 g
Sugar: 2 g

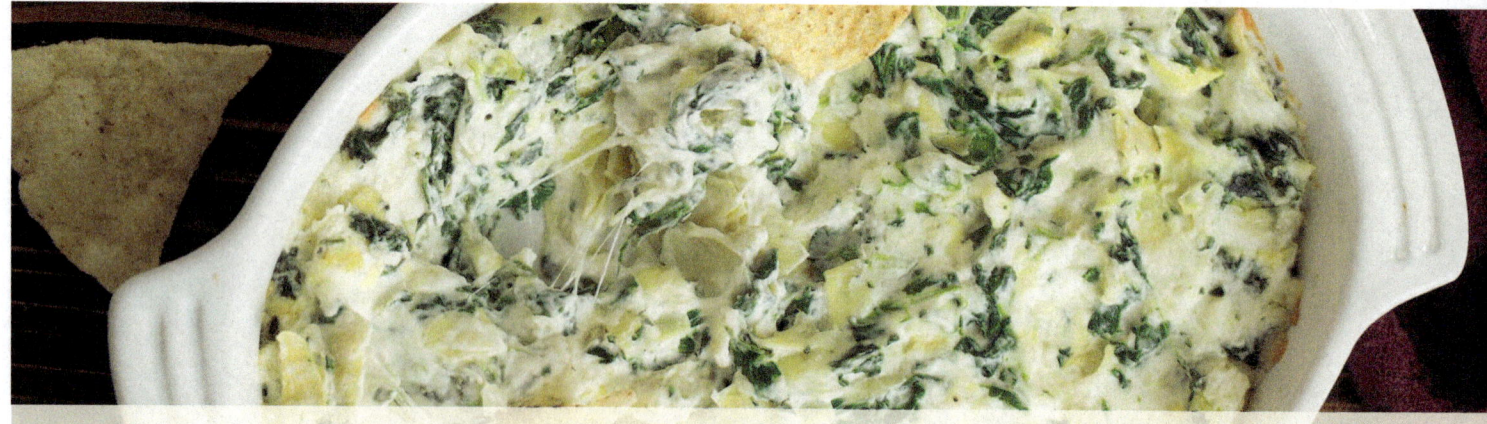

CREAMY SPINACH AND ARTICHOKE DIP

Creamy Spinach and Artichoke Dip is a rich and flavorful appetizer that combines tender spinach, artichoke hearts, and a creamy blend of cheeses. It's perfect for serving at parties or enjoying as a hearty snack with your favorite dippers.

Serves 	Preparation Time	Cooking Time 
4	10 minutes	30 minute

Ingredients:

1 (10 oz) package frozen chopped spinach, thawed and drained
1 (14 oz) can artichoke hearts, drained and chopped
1 cup sour cream
1 cup mayonnaise
1 cup grated Parmesan cheese
1 cup shredded mozzarella cheese
2 cloves garlic, minced
1/4 teaspoon salt
1/4 teaspoon black pepper
1/4 teaspoon crushed red pepper flakes (optional, for a bit of heat)

Instructions:

1. **Preheat Oven:** Preheat your oven to 375°F (190°C).
2. **Prepare the Dip Mixture:** In a large mixing bowl, combine the chopped spinach, artichoke hearts, sour cream, mayonnaise, Parmesan cheese, mozzarella cheese, minced garlic, salt, pepper, and crushed red pepper flakes (if using). Mix until well combined.
3. **Transfer and Bake:** Transfer the mixture to a baking dish (an 8x8-inch dish or a similar size works well).Smooth the top with a spatula.
4. **Bake the Dip:** Bake in the preheated oven for 25-30 minutes, or until the dip is hot and bubbly, and the top is golden brown.
5. **Serve:** Allow the dip to cool slightly before serving.Serve warm with tortilla chips, pita bread, crackers, or fresh vegetable sticks for dipping.

Nutrients (per serving)

Calories: 220 Sodium: 450 mg Carbohydrates: 8 g
Fiber: 2 g Protein: 10 g Calcium: 250 mg Fat: 18 g
Sugar: 2 g

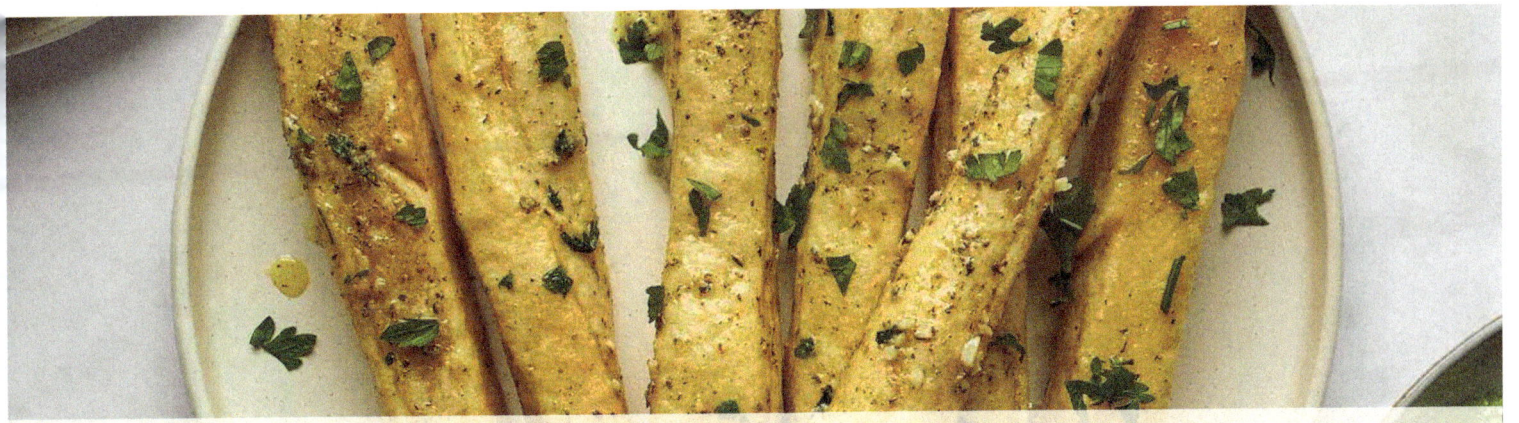

GARLIC BREADSTICKS

Garlic Breadsticks are a classic and irresistible side dish that complements any meal. They are soft, buttery, and infused with garlic flavor, making them a favorite for dipping in marinara sauce or enjoying on their own.

Serves 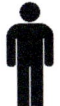	Preparation Time	Cooking Time 
4	20 minutes	15 minute

Ingredients:

1 1/2 cups warm water (110°F/45°C)
1 tablespoon sugar
2 1/4 teaspoons (1 packet) active dry yeast
3 1/2 to 4 cups all-purpose flour
1/4 cup olive oil
1 teaspoon salt
4 tablespoons unsalted butter, melted
4 cloves garlic, minced
2 tablespoons chopped fresh parsley (or 2 teaspoons dried parsley)
1/4 teaspoon garlic powder (optional, for extra garlic flavor)
1/4 teaspoon dried oregano (optional)

Instructions:

1. **Prepare the Dough:** In a small bowl, combine warm water and sugar. Sprinkle yeast over the water and let it sit for about 5 minutes, or until frothy. In a large bowl, mix 3 1/2 cups of flour and salt. Make a well in the center and pour in the yeast mixture and olive oil. Stir until a dough forms. If the dough is too sticky, gradually add more flour, 1 tablespoon at a time, until it becomes soft and elastic.
2. **Knead the Dough:** Transfer the dough to a floured surface and knead for about 5-7 minutes, or until smooth and elastic. Place the dough in a lightly oiled bowl, cover with a damp cloth or plastic wrap, and let it rise in a warm place for about 1 hour, or until doubled in size.
3. **Prepare the Breadsticks:** Preheat your oven to 400°F (200°C). Punch down the risen dough and transfer it to a floured surface. Roll the dough out into a rectangle about 1/2-inch thick. Cut the dough into strips about 1/2 inch wide and transfer them to a parchment-lined baking sheet.
4. **Add Garlic and Herbs:** In a small bowl, mix the melted butter, minced garlic, parsley, garlic powder (if using), and dried oregano (if using). Brush the garlic butter mixture generously over the breadsticks.
5. **Bake:** Bake in the preheated oven for 12-15 minutes, or until the breadsticks are golden brown.
6. **Serve:** Serve warm. Enjoy with marinara sauce, Alfredo sauce, or on its own.

Nutrients (per serving)

Calories: 120 Sodium: 180 mg Carbohydrates: 18 g
Fiber: 1 g Protein: 3 g Calcium: 15 mg Fat: 4 g
Sugar: 2 g

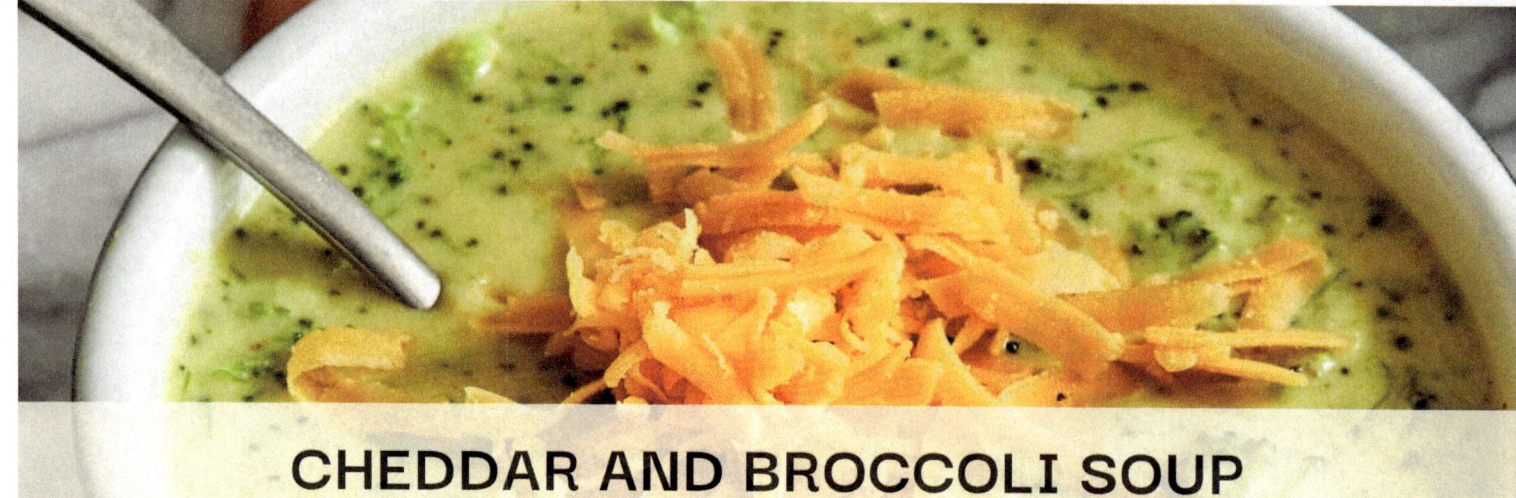

CHEDDAR AND BROCCOLI SOUP

Cheddar and Broccoli Soup is a comforting, creamy dish that combines the earthy flavors of broccoli with the rich, sharp taste of cheddar cheese. This soup is perfect for a cozy lunch or dinner, especially when paired with crusty bread.

Serves		Preparation Time		Cooking Time	
4		15 minutes		25 minute	

Ingredients:

4 cups broccoli florets
1 small onion, diced
2 cloves garlic, minced
4 tablespoons unsalted butter
4 tablespoons all-purpose flour
4 cups low-sodium chicken or vegetable broth
2 cups whole milk
1 cup heavy cream
2 cups sharp cheddar cheese, shredded
1/2 teaspoon mustard powder (optional)
Salt and pepper to taste
1/4 teaspoon ground nutmeg (optional)
1/2 cup grated Parmesan cheese (optional, for garnish)

Instructions:

1. **Cook the Broccoli:** In a large pot, bring lightly salted water to a boil. Add the broccoli florets and cook for 3-4 minutes, until just tender. Drain and set aside.
2. **Sauté the Onion and Garlic:** In the same pot, melt the butter over medium heat. Add the diced onion and sauté for 3-4 minutes, until softened. Add the minced garlic and sauté for another minute.
3. **Make the Roux:** Sprinkle the flour over the onions and garlic, stirring constantly to make a roux. Cook for 2-3 minutes, until the mixture turns a light golden color.
4. **Add the Liquids:** Gradually whisk in the broth, making sure there are no lumps. Then, whisk in the milk and cream. Bring the mixture to a simmer and cook for 5-7 minutes, until slightly thickened.
5. **Combine and Season:** Add the cooked broccoli to the pot. Using an immersion blender, blend the soup until smooth (or leave some broccoli chunks if you prefer a chunkier texture). Stir in the shredded cheddar cheese until fully melted. Add mustard powder, salt, pepper, and nutmeg, adjusting the seasoning to taste.
6. **Serve:** Ladle the soup into bowls and, if desired, garnish with grated Parmesan cheese. Serve hot with crusty bread or crackers.

Nutrients (per serving)

Calories: 350 Sodium: 400 mg Carbohydrates: 15 g
Fiber: 2 g Protein: 12 g Calcium: 250 mg Fat: 28 g
Sugar: 6 g

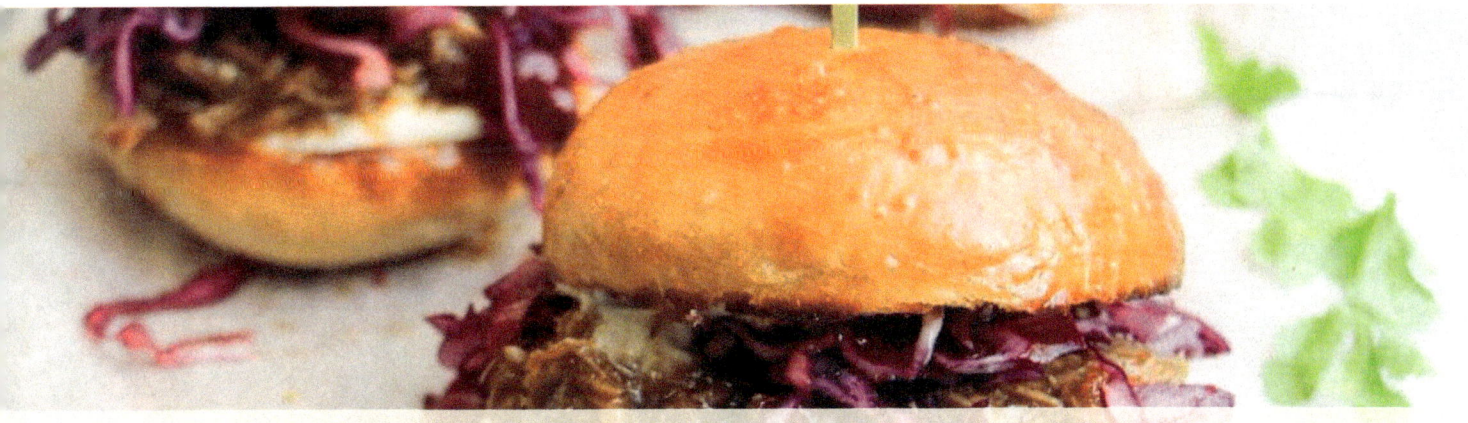

BBQ PULLED PORK SLIDERS

BBQ Pulled Pork Sliders are a delicious and satisfying dish perfect for any gathering or casual meal. Slow-cooked to tender perfection and coated in a rich BBQ sauce, the pulled pork is served on soft slider buns, making it a crowd-pleasing favorite.

Serves	Preparation Time	Cooking Time
4	15 minutes	8-10 hours

Ingredients:

2 lbs pork shoulder (or pork butt)
1 large onion, sliced
3 cloves garlic, minced
1 cup BBQ sauce (your favorite brand)
1/2 cup chicken broth
2 tablespoons apple cider vinegar
1 tablespoon brown sugar
1 teaspoon smoked paprika
1 teaspoon chili powder
1 teaspoon cumin
Salt and pepper to taste
12 slider buns
Coleslaw (optional, for topping)

Instructions:

1. **Prepare the Pork:** Rub the pork shoulder with smoked paprika, chili powder, cumin, salt, and pepper. Ensure the spices are evenly distributed over the meat.
2. **Slow Cook the Pork:** Place the sliced onion and minced garlic in the bottom of a slow cooker. Place the seasoned pork shoulder on top. Pour the chicken broth and apple cider vinegar over the pork. Cook on low for 8-10 hours, or on high for 4-6 hours, until the pork is tender and easily shredded.
3. **Shred the Pork:** Once cooked, remove the pork from the slow cooker and shred it using two forks. Discard any excess fat. Return the shredded pork to the slow cooker and mix it with the cooking juices.
4. **Add the BBQ Sauce:** Stir in the BBQ sauce and brown sugar. Let the pork cook on low for an additional 30 minutes to absorb the flavors.
5. **Assemble the Sliders:** Slice the slider buns in half. Place a generous portion of BBQ pulled pork on the bottom half of each bun. If desired, top with coleslaw for added crunch and flavor. Place the top half of the bun over the filling.
6. **Serve:** Serve the sliders warm, with extra BBQ sauce on the side if desired.

Nutrients (per serving)

Calories: 320 Sodium: 600 mg Carbohydrates: 32 g
Fiber: 2 g Protein: 18 g Calcium: 50 mg Fat: 15 g
Sugar: 10 g

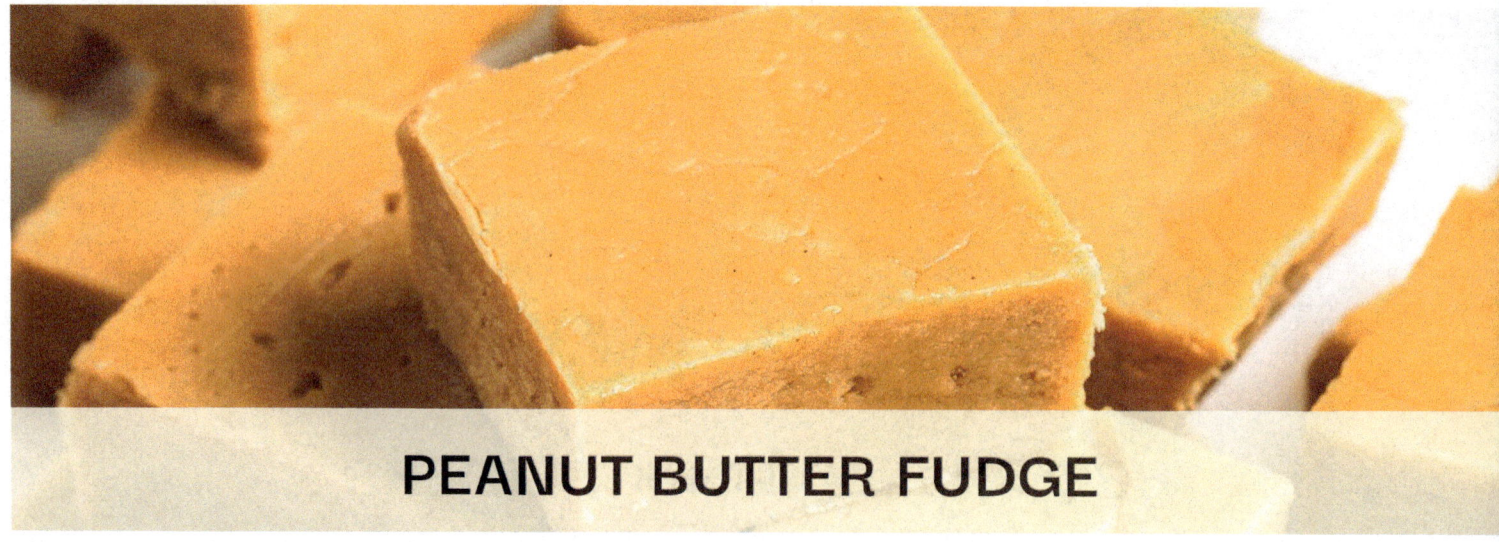

PEANUT BUTTER FUDGE

Peanut Butter Fudge is a rich, creamy treat that's perfect for satisfying your sweet tooth. Made with just a few simple ingredients, this fudge is a quick and easy dessert that everyone will love.

Serves 	Preparation Time	Cooking Time 
4	10 minutes	1.5 hour

Ingredients:

2 cups granulated sugar
1/2 cup unsalted butter
1/2 cup whole milk
1 cup creamy peanut butter
1 teaspoon vanilla extract
1/4 teaspoon salt

Could add Sultanas Walnuts

Instructions:

1. **Prepare the Pan:** Line an 8x8-inch baking pan with parchment paper, leaving some overhang on the sides for easy removal later.
2. **Cook the Sugar Mixture:** In a medium saucepan, combine the sugar, butter and milk. Cook over medium heat, stirring constantly until the mixture comes to a boil. Continue boiling for 2-3 minutes, stirring frequently to prevent burning.
3. **Add the Peanut Butter:** Remove the saucepan from heat. Stir in the peanut butter, vanilla extract, and salt until the mixture is smooth and well combined.
4. **Pour and Set:** Quickly pour the peanut butter mixture into the prepared baking pan, spreading it evenly with a spatula. Let it cool at room temperature for about 30 minutes, then refrigerate for at least 1 hour until the fudge is firm.
5. **Cut and Serve:** Once set, lift the fudge out of the pan using the parchment paper overhang. Cut it into small squares and serve.

Nutrients (per serving)

Calories: 150 Sodium: 45 mg Carbohydrates: 19 g
Fiber: 1 g Protein: 2 g Calcium: 5 mg Fat: 8 g
Sugar: 18 g

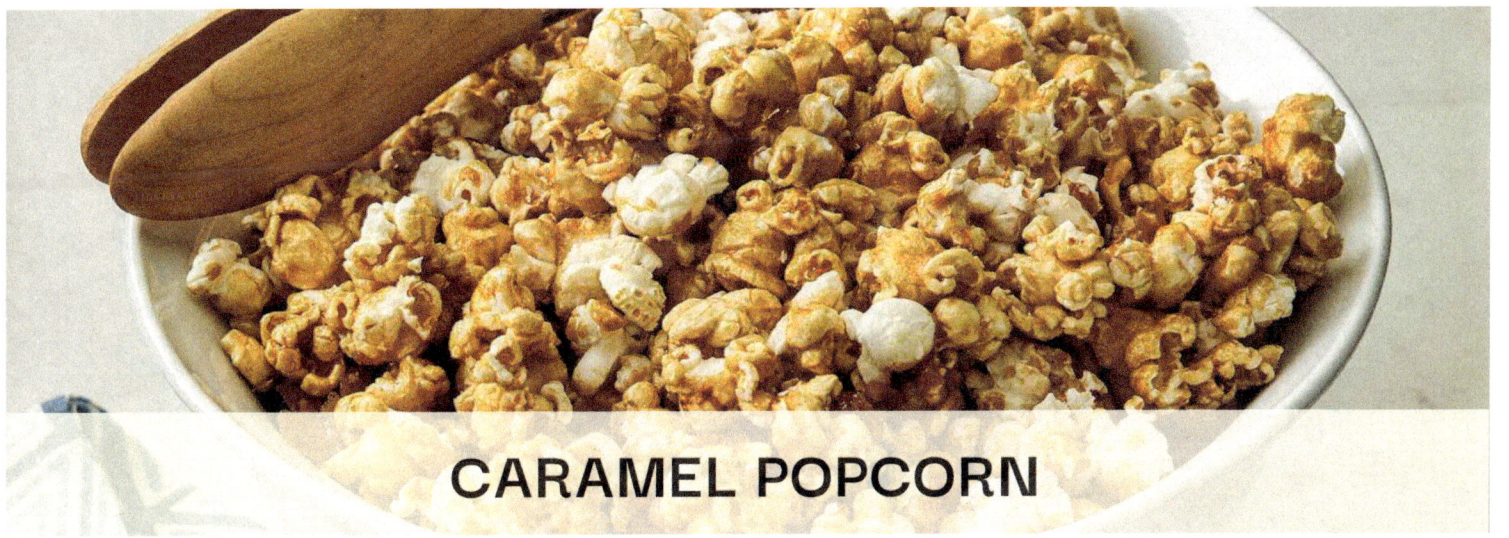

CARAMEL POPCORN

Caramel Popcorn is a delicious, crunchy treat that's perfect for movie nights, parties, or simply satisfying your sweet cravings. The combination of buttery caramel and light, airy popcorn makes for an irresistible snack.

Serves	Preparation Time	Cooking Time
4	15 minutes	1 hour

Ingredients:

10 cups popped popcorn (about 1/2 cup unpopped kernels)
1 cup unsalted butter
1 cup brown sugar, packed
1/4 cup light corn syrup
1/2 teaspoon salt
1/2 teaspoon baking soda
1 teaspoon vanilla extract

Instructions:

1. **Prepare the Popcorn:** Pop the popcorn using an air popper or stovetop method. Transfer the popcorn to a large bowl, making sure to remove any unpopped kernels.
2. **Make the Caramel Sauce:** In a medium saucepan, melt the butter over medium heat. Add the brown sugar, corn syrup, and salt. Stir until the mixture is fully combined. Bring the mixture to a boil, stirring constantly. Once boiling, stop stirring and let it cook for 4-5 minutes without disturbing it. The caramel should reach a deep amber color.
3. **Add Baking Soda and Vanilla:** Remove the caramel from heat. Quickly stir in the baking soda and vanilla extract. The mixture will foam up slightly; stir until smooth.
4. **Coat the Popcorn:** Pour the hot caramel over the popcorn. Using a spatula, gently toss the popcorn to evenly coat it with the caramel.
5. **Bake for Crispiness:** Preheat your oven to 250°F (120°C). Spread the caramel-coated popcorn onto a large baking sheet lined with parchment paper. Bake the popcorn for 45-60 minutes, stirring every 15 minutes to ensure even coating and crispiness.
6. **Cool and Serve:** Once baked, remove the popcorn from the oven and let it cool completely on the baking sheet. Break it into clusters and serve or store in an airtight container.

Nutrients (per serving)

Calories: 150 Sodium: 100 mg Carbohydrates: 24 g
Fiber: 1 g Protein: 1 g Calcium: 10 mg Fat: 7 g
Sugar: 18 g

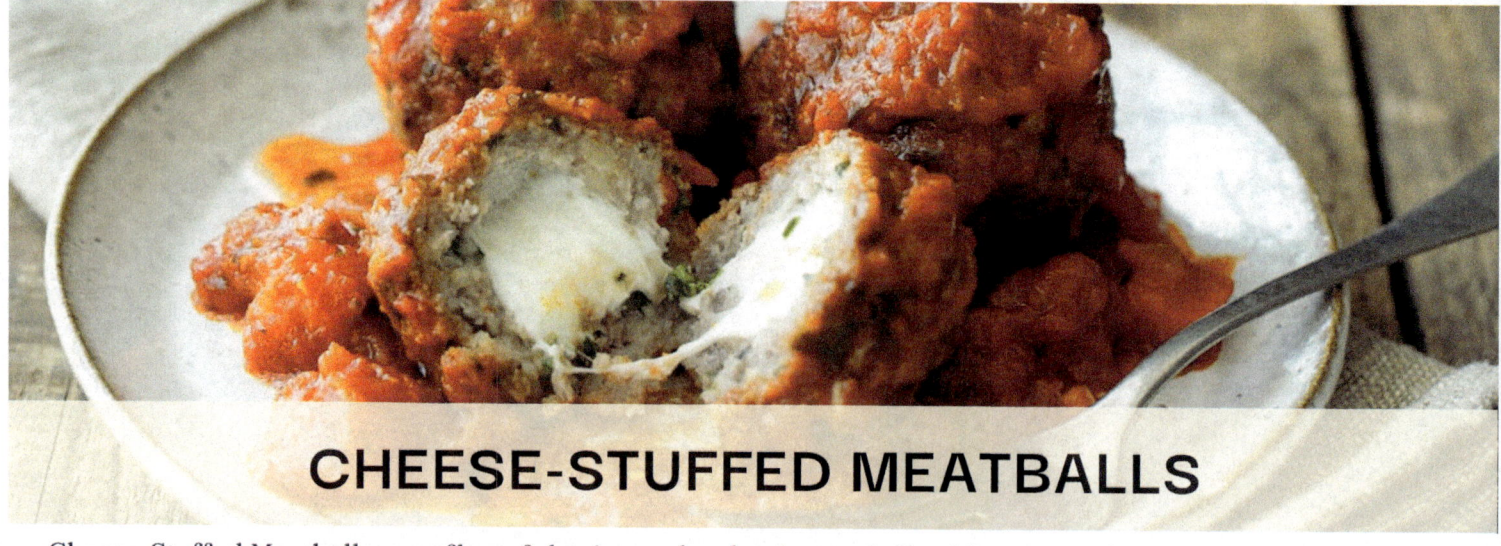

CHEESE-STUFFED MEATBALLS

Cheese-Stuffed Meatballs are a flavorful twist on the classic meatball, with a gooey cheese surprise in the center. These meatballs are perfect for appetizers, a main course, or even as a filling for sandwiches.

Serves 	Preparation Time	Cooking Time 
4	20 minutes	20 minute

Ingredients:

1 lb ground beef (80% lean)
1/2 lb ground pork
1/2 cup breadcrumbs
1/4 cup grated Parmesan cheese
1/4 cup milk
1 large egg
2 cloves garlic, minced
1 tablespoon chopped fresh parsley
1 teaspoon salt
1/2 teaspoon black pepper
1/2 teaspoon dried oregano
4 oz mozzarella cheese, cut into small cubes
2 tablespoons olive oil (for cooking)

Instructions:

1. **Prepare the Meat Mixture:** In a large mixing bowl, combine the ground beef, ground pork, breadcrumbs, Parmesan cheese, milk, egg, minced garlic, parsley, salt, pepper, and oregano. Mix until all the ingredients are evenly distributed.
2. **Form the Meatballs:** Take a small portion of the meat mixture (about 2 tablespoons) and flatten it in your hand. Place a cube of mozzarella cheese in the center, then fold the meat around the cheese, rolling it into a ball. Repeat with the remaining meat mixture and cheese cubes.
3. **Cook the Meatballs:** Heat olive oil in a large skillet over medium heat. Once the oil is hot, add the meatballs, making sure not to overcrowd the pan. Cook the meatballs for 4-5 minutes on each side, or until they are browned all over and cooked through. The internal temperature should reach 160°F (70°C).
4. **Serve:** Remove the meatballs from the skillet and let them rest for a few minutes. Serve them hot with your favorite sauce, pasta, or as part of a meatball sub.

Nutrients (per serving)

Calories: 290 Sodium: 500 mg Carbohydrates: 5 g
Fiber: 0 g Protein: 24 g Calcium: 120 mg Fat: 20 g
Sugar: 1 g

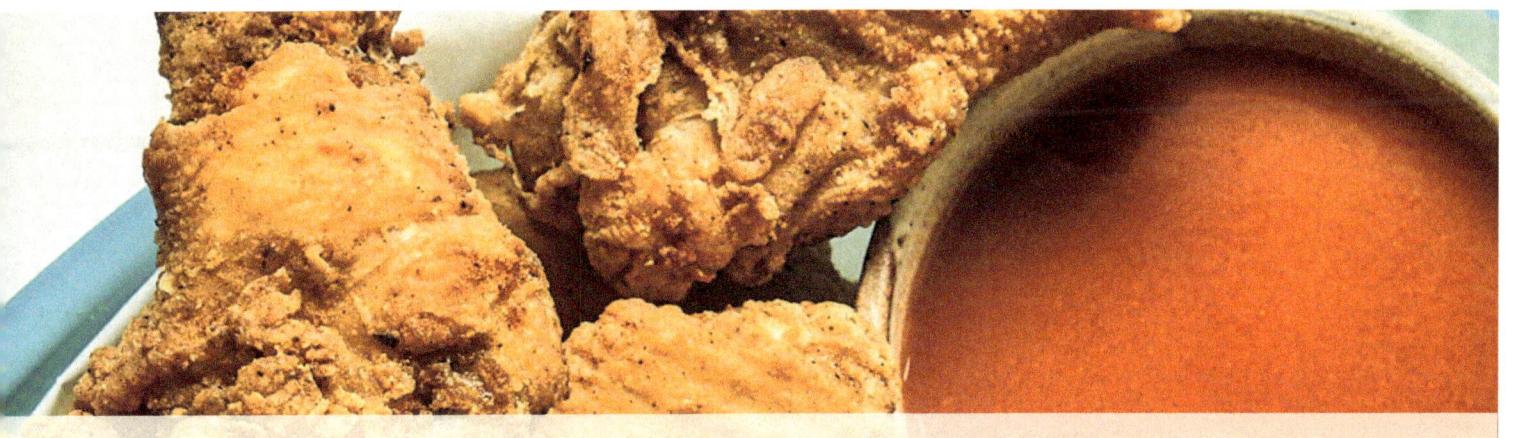

FRIED CHICKEN WINGS

Fried Chicken Wings are a classic favorite, known for their crispy exterior and juicy, tender meat. Perfect for game days, parties, or a comforting snack, these wings are sure to be a hit with everyone.

Serves 	Preparation Time	Cooking Time 
4	15 minutes	20 minute

Ingredients:

2 lbs chicken wings, split at the joint, tips removed
1 cup all-purpose flour
1/2 cup cornstarch
1 tablespoon garlic powder
1 tablespoon onion powder
1 teaspoon paprika
1 teaspoon salt
1/2 teaspoon black pepper
1/2 teaspoon cayenne pepper (optional for heat)
1 cup buttermilk
Vegetable oil for frying

Instructions:

1. **Prepare the Wings:** Rinse and pat dry the chicken wings with paper towels. Place them in a large bowl and pour the buttermilk over the wings, ensuring they are well coated. Let the wings marinate in the buttermilk for at least 30 minutes, or up to 4 hours in the refrigerator.
2. **Coat the Wings:** In a shallow dish, combine the flour, cornstarch, garlic powder, onion powder, paprika, salt, black pepper, and cayenne pepper. Mix well.Remove the wings from the buttermilk, letting any excess drip off. Dredge each wing in the flour mixture, pressing lightly to ensure an even coating. Place the coated wings on a plate or baking sheet.
3. **Fry the Wings:** Heat about 2 inches of vegetable oil in a deep skillet or Dutch oven to 350°F (175°C).Carefully add the wings to the hot oil in batches, being careful not to overcrowd the pan. Fry the wings for 8-10 minutes, turning occasionally, until they are golden brown and crispy. The internal temperature should reach 165°F (74°C).Use a slotted spoon to remove the wings from the oil, placing them on a paper towel-lined plate to drain any excess oil.
4. **Serve:** Serve the fried chicken wings hot, with your choice of dipping sauces such as ranch, blue cheese, or barbecue sauce.

Nutrients (per serving)

Calories: 420 Sodium: 550 mg Carbohydrates: 18 g
Fiber: 1 g Protein: 25 g Calcium: 40 mg Fat: 28 g
Sugar: 1 g

Printed in Great Britain
by Amazon